PROBIOTICS
NATURE'S INTERNAL HEALERS

"Anyone interested in their body ecology,
will want to have this book
in their library."

Dr. Earl Mindell
Best-selling author of
Earl Mindell's Vitamin Bible

PROBIOTICS
NATURE'S INTERNAL HEALERS

NATASHA TRENEV

Avery Publishing Group
Garden City Park, New York

616.014
T794
c.1 P1

The information in this book is based on the training, personal experiences, and research of the author. It is intended for educational purposes, and is not meant to diagnose, prescribe, or replace medical care. Mention of any research organization or individual researcher should in no way be construed as an endorsement of this book or of any of the techniques therein. Because each person and situation are unique, the author and publisher urge the reader to check with a qualified health professional before using any procedure in which there is any question to appropriateness. It is a sign of wisdom, not cowardice, to seek a second or third opinion.

The publisher does not advocate the use of any particular health treatment, but believes the information presented in this book should be available to the public.

Cover Design: William Gonzalez
Typesetter: Elaine V. McCaw
In-House Editor: Marie Caratozzolo
Printer: Paragon Press, Honesdale, PA

Avery Publishing Group
120 Old Broadway
Garden City Park, NY 11040
1-800-548-5757

Cataloging-in-Publication Data

Trenev, Natasha
        Probiotics : nature's internal healers / by Natasha Trenev.
                p.   cm.
        Includes bibliographical references and index.
        ISBN 0–89529–847–3
        1. Intestines—Microbiology.   2. Microorganisms—Therapeutic
use.
        I. Title.
        QR171.I6T74   1998
        616' .014—dc21   98–11979
                                                                                    CIP

Contents

PART TWO — THE DISORDERS

General Guidelines for Taking Probiotics,   137

*I dedicate this book to my devoted husband and daughter
whose love and support have made all of my endeavors possible,
and to the spiritual belief that teaches me
that work done in the spirit of service to humanity
is accounted as worshiping God.*

Acknowledgments

I would like to acknowledge my professional admiration for Randy Porubcan, a great fellow enthusiast for probiotics and the CEO of Advanced Microbial Systems—a company that manufactures highest-quality soil and environmental probiotics; for Dr. Michael McCann, a great humanitarian and the best family doctor of any age; for Dr. Hobel and Dr. Greenspoon of Cedars-Sinai Medical Center at Los Angeles, who have given freely of their time to advance the cause of probiotics in the medical arena; for John Booth, a tireless and devoted promoter of probiotics in Australia; and, finally, for Marie Caratozzolo, my editor at Avery, who is a joy to work with on any level.

Foreword

Probiotics will be to medicine in the twenty-first century as antibiotics and microbiology were in the twentieth. Physicians on the front line of medical practice increasingly recognize the limitations and complications of conventional approaches of medical practices, only one of which is the overuse of antibiotics. In this book, Natasha Trenev makes a compelling case that probiotics should be recognized not only for a wide variety of practical uses, but also as a legitimate specialty worthy of the best methods of scientific inquiry.

Predating modern medicine, probiotics is just being rediscovered by modern medical scientists, even though diseases of antiquity were benefited by this science. It is an honor, then, to introduce the reader to this pioneer of medicine, who is exploring new territory much like the great explorers of past frontiers—including Galileo, Columbus, Leewenhouk and Pasteur—have done in their fields.

"Pro" meaning "for" or "in favor of," "biotics" or "life" aptly describes this new/old method. It contrasts directly with "anti" "biotics" or "killing life." It means giving live friendly bacteria to a patient to maintain or restore health. Long recognized in the animal feed business, friendly or beneficial bacterial supplements are routinely used because increased weight and healthier animals mean increased profits. We know that domestic animals suffer the same diseases as humans, yet we have been slow to recognize and adapt these methods for ourselves. Recently, in an effort to prevent *Salmonella* disease in chickens, the FDA has approved the use of probiotics in a multibacterial spray. Newborn chicks are coated with the spray, then, as they peck at their feathers, they ingest the friendly bacteria, which take up residence in their intestinal tracts, preventing harmful microbes from taking root.

Government and organized medicine have often impeded those pioneers who advocate probiotic use in humans. Rather than provide help and encouragement, they have often impeded these forerunners by restricting or interfering with their advocacy of probiotics for specific diseases in humans. Thankfully, the field was well established in the food supplement area long before the FDA was even a thought. Even though the government has a role in protecting the public health by insuring the quality of products, they should let the natural laws of scientific inquiry sort out fact from fiction.

A personal experience is worth mentioning here. For many years, I agonized with my patients who suffered from inflammatory bowel disease (ulcerative colitis or Crohn's disease). I believed there had to be better treatment methods than mutilating surgery or toxic drugs like corticosteroids. There were some clinical clues that the basic problem was a disturbance in the normal bowel flora. For example, in many cases, the disease was initiated or precipitated after a course of antibiotics. In some of these cases, an overgrowth of certain toxic anaerobic bacteria called *Clostridia* were found to be the culprits, but in most cases, the cause could not be found. On the other hand, some longstanding severe cases were temporarily "cured" by combinations of antimicrobials. As soon as the antibiotics were discontinued, the disease inevitably recurred. So how could the same treatment cause opposite results—exacerbations in some and cures in others? It's easy if one understands the principles of probiotics.

Let's take your front lawn as an example. If you killed off all of the grass with a powerful herbicide (akin to antibiotic effects on the gastrointestinal flora) and then waited, what would you get? Not a nice mono-crop of "beneficial" grasses, but a variety of weeds that you do not want. Now, instead of waiting for nature to take its course (as we routinely do in medical practice), let's say you reseeded with large numbers of beneficial grass seeds. Now you would expect a lovely mono-crop, or better yet, a mixture of beneficial strains. This actually happened to me in 1963 when I tried to save money by reseeding a lawn with a stingy amount of seeds. I got mostly weeds, until I reseeded with a much larger number of seeds. Then I had a lovely lawn.

Maybe this was a good experience for me because I was reminded of this long-forgotten suburban experiment in groundskeeping when Natasha Trenev called me to say, "Of course your patients relapse when you stop giving the beneficial bacteria. You have to keep giving them!"

"Well, baloney," was my initial reaction. Everyone knows the bowel flora establishes itself early in life and is very resistant to change. But her idea nagged at me—maybe, just maybe, she was right. On my very next two patients, one who suffered from Crohn's disease, and the other from ulcerative colitis, my colleagues and I continued giving them beneficial bacteria after treatment was completed. Unlike previous patients, these two stayed in remission and both continue to have normal colon biopsies.

In the early 1970s, I had one patient—a teenager—who had long suffered from bloody bowel movements that were increasing in frequency and intensity. He had become anemic, had lost weight, and had stopped growing. Barium x-ray examination revealed severe ulcerative colitis. Another patient—an elderly man in his seventies—suffering from Crohn's disease, had had consultations at the Mayo Clinic and the University of Chicago, where surgical removal of his large bowel and rectum was recommended. In both cases, following broad-spectrum decontamination of the existing gastrointestinal bacteria, these patients were given an entirely new bowel flora.

The teenager enjoyed good health and complete remission for the next fifteen years. I was certain that he was cured, but after all those years, he relapsed, and before I knew it, he had had a colectomy (surgical removal of part of the large intestine). What had happened? Presumably, his abnormal bowel flora had gradually reestablished itself, but there was no proof of this, only speculation. The next few patients relapsed much sooner. Something had gone wrong.

The elderly patient, on the other hand, did not relapse. We discovered that on his own initiative, he had continued to take a daily supplement of *L. acidophilus*. Enter Natasha Trenev. She seized on this clue and encouraged us to continue supplementing our patients with these normal, helpful bacteria. Since then, none of our patients have relapsed. It will take many years to prove that her insights are correct, but I, for one, am sure she is right. Remember the reseeded lawn? Unless we reseed the bare spots, the weeds will gradually take over.

Most physicians not only ignored this approach in treating Crohn's disease and ileitis, they ridiculed it. How could an obscure pediatrician who is not even in the "club," and a non-physician like Natasha Trenev find so simple a cure for these two disabling diseases in some of these patients? How is it possible that they could provide answers to questions that had eluded the best minds in medicine for over a century?

Others, however, like Dr. Robert A. Good of the University of South Florida, encouraged me. Dr. Robert P. Nelson also offered helpful criticisms, as did Drs. Martin Klemperer, Mandel Sher, Sami Bahna, Roberto Nicolo, Krishna Urval, all of those involved in Dr. Good's department of Immunology at All Children's Hospital in St. Petersburg, Florida, and Robert Buck in Cleveland, Ohio. One American physician, Dr. J. D. Bennet, bravely performed a similar recolonization procedure on himself, and Dr. Richard Abrams of Chicago, Illinois, successfully treated his own son.

For the most part, European, Scandinavian, and Australian physicians' attitudes are far ahead of ours here in the States. For example, there are thirteen different companies in Germany alone who sell friendly species of *E. coli* bacteria over-the-counter without a prescription. In the United States—none.

During the cold war in Europe, when there was a paucity of money for medicines, one creative Czechoslovakian pediatrician, Dr. R. Zadnikova, used a probiotic mixture of a facultative anaerobic lactobacillus along with a benign *E. coli* to prevent hospital acquired infections in newborns. Her results were highly significant. This very effective and inexpensive treatment, administered by mouth immediately after birth, almost completely prevented diseases such as necrotizing enterocolitis and sepsis. This approach was particularly effective in cesarean section births. In the United States, where we blast away with a broader and broader spectrum of antibiotics, this idea is anathema. "McCann," I was challenged, "you are actually advocating feeding fecal flora to our newborns?" Well, yes, in a manner of speaking. How do you think the normal baby acquires his normal gastrointestinal flora? From his mother, that's where. And more specifically, from his mother's normal healthy (or unhealthy) vaginal flora. Where do you think the baby who is born by cesarean section gets his? From anywhere in the nursery—often hospital pathogens carried by unsuspecting and well-meaning nursery personnel, most often doctors and nurses. We have interfered with many thousands of years of natural selection of the most beneficial symbiotic hosts of man—the normal gastrointestinal flora.

We might easily remedy this situation by adopting health-promoting practices of probiotics, although this will require re-education of both the general public and our medical policy makers—no easy task. The challenge is made more formidable, when, for example, *E.coli* is considered synonymous with evil disease, and only a tiny minority make the distinction between "good" and "bad" *E. coli*. There is in our society deeply ingrained fear of bacteria and the infectious diseases associated with them. We drench our foods in preservatives and wash our hands with antibacterial soap. These fears are, of course, somewhat warranted—as the recent highly publicized cases of beef contaminated with a bad strain of *E. coli* demonstrates—but they make the task of education all the more daunting. It is no wonder then that very few people, including heath professionals, realize that all *E. coli* are not created equal. As with many other species of animals, *E. coli* includes distinct strains that can kill us, and other strains that can defend us from virulent invaders.

Thankfully, lactobacilli and bifidobacteria species, the two predominant normal flora of the upper and lower gastrointestinal tract, have acquired good connotations, neither having been associated with disease. Streptococcus is another normal inhabitant that has mixed, mostly bad, connotations. That is why this book is so refreshing and important. It tackles directly these societal taboos, and challenges us in the scientific medical community to ask these new questions: Can we attach antigens to these bacteria that will stimulate natural immunity to contagious diseases? Can we treat or, better yet, prevent autoimmune diseases like rheumatoid arthritis, ankylosing spondylitis, Crohn's disease, ulcerative colitis, and many others in which antigens of the gut or joint epithelium are shared or identical to those of the bacteria in the normal gastrointestinal flora? Can we prevent certain cancers? The evidence is compelling. The answer to all of these questions appears to be yes.

Nonetheless, certain caution is warranted. I do not mean to endorse all of the claims put forth in this book. As this is a relatively new field, many of the conclusions are necessarily based on testimonials and anecdote. We know that testimonials can lead to conclusions derived erroneously from accidental, but not causal, associations. And yet, case histories cannot be ignored or dismissed without carefully controlled and blinded prospective analyses.

These cases should be the fertile ground for the eager young scientists of the twenty-first century, just like the great minds of the twentieth century tackled individual microbes—polio, streptococcus, pneumoccoccus, clostridium tetanus, and many others. Only now we have the challenge of the role of each in the interaction of multiple species to establish dominance, considering that 400 different known species of individual bacteria, not to mention viruses and parasites, inhabit the normal bowel. If any one individual has five or ten individual species of microorganisms, each fighting to maintain its niche, and any other individual has five or ten other entirely different species, all fighting to maintain their own niches, then one can imagine the complexity. (Add to this the fact that many of these species have yet to be identified.) It will take computers and minds more creative than mine to put all of this together. Meanwhile, microbes—the largest bio-mass on earth—continue to mutate against man's antibiotics and other weapons, and to assert their place, oblivious to the cares of *Homo sapiens*.

I applaud the courage of Natasha Trenev to challenge the imagination of a new generation of scientific pioneers and explorers in this vast new continent of ideas. Not since Columbus' discovery of America has such an opportunity for brave new explorers presented itself. Let us begin.

Michael L. McCann, M.D.
Cleveland, Ohio

Probiotics: Nature's Internal Healers

Introduction

*I*n any day and age, there will always be people who make an effort to learn what they need to know to survive and thrive in their environment. Considering the state of the world today, there is a great need for authoritative information on self-care health care. There are no innocent bystanders. The quality of health that you enjoy—good or bad—depends, to a large extent, on how much you know and how well you take care of yourself and those you love. This book will tell you what you need to know.

NOW HEAR THIS

Your intestinal tract is home to around 100 trillion microorganisms, and not all of them are friendly. Some of the most dangerous offenders enter your body in the food you eat, the water you drink, and the air you breathe. These microorganisms are so small they are invisible to the naked eye, and there is no way to keep them out. Many of these bacteria are mere nuisances. Some might make you sick for a few days, while others can make you miserably ill for months. Still others carry infectious diseases that doctors are finding increasingly difficult to treat effectively. The worst of these microorganisms can be deadly.

No matter where you live, there is no escape. Once dangerous bacteria enter your body, the fight is on. Your body must deal with these microbes as best it can. Often the body does a good job of handling alien invaders, but sometimes it is just not well enough equipped to fight and win the battles that are continually waged, minute-by-minute, day after day, year after year. Your bacterial enemies are never vanquished once and for all; the battles are never-ending. You eat, you drink, and you breathe. And, with every bite, every swallow, and every breath—during every second of your life—you take in billions and billions of bacteria. These wars with bacteria go on as long as you live.

Unfriendly microorganisms come in many guises. Some are easily identified disease carriers. Others are chameleons, harmless at times, harmful at others. They can be neutral under certain conditions, but—like *Candida albicans*, the inoffensive yeast that can turn into a predatory and dangerous fungus—they can also become decidedly unfriendly when they proliferate and spread to take over formerly friendly held territories. Opportunistic organisms that turn foe create problems by causing an infection themselves and/or by aiding and abetting the disease-causing organisms that seek a home in your gastrointestinal tract.

THE PROBLEM

You've probably been hearing a great deal about the problems facing the medical profession today. Television news shows, books, and newspaper and magazine articles cite frightening statistics about the incurable bacterial and viral diseases surfacing around the globe. This is not a distant phenomenon specific to countries on the other side of the world. The World Health Organization (WHO) warns that any microbe—good, bad, or ugly—can make its way around the world in forty-eight hours. In addition, some familiar diseases—including staph and strep infections, pneumonia, tuberculosis, meningitis, and malaria—which were once easily treated, may not necessarily be so any longer. Today, even when doctors resort to the strongest weapons in their arsenals, many of these "wonder drugs" don't work as effectively as they once did.

It was in the late 1920s that Alexander Fleming discovered penicillin. By the early 1950s, this "miracle medicine" was readily available, and doctors were using it against all sorts of bacterial diseases and infections. Penicillin and its derivatives knocked out pneumonia and other dreaded diseases easily. The "bad bugs" didn't stand a chance. With the advent of penicillin, a whole new category of drugs dubbed antibiotics came into being. This compound word comes from the Greek *anti* (against) and *biotics* (life). Simply put, antibiotics kill living bacteria.

Antibiotics were designed to destroy a wide range of the dangerous infectious organisms that make you sick. Drug companies competed with one another to get in on this lucrative market. More and more antibiotics were rushed into development, and they all worked wonderfully well. When antibiotics were ingested or injected, the bad bacteria were destroyed and the patient recovered.

By the 1970s, most of the medical detectives began to rest on their laurels. It appeared that antibiotics could cure just about anything. Pharmaceutical scientists were sure that there was no longer any reason to continue with the intense research and development of drugs that had characterized the previous decades. For one thing, it was costly and time-consuming. To bring a new drug to market, the cost could be as high as $300 million dollars and the process could take up to five years. The more important reason, however, was that health authorities believed the job was done. They felt assured that by the year 2000, infectious diseases would be gone forever.

Unfortunately, they were wrong. Today, more than 19,000 people die every year from untreatable diseases caused by drug-resistant bacteria that continue to thrive even when attacked by the most powerful antibiotics. Newer antibiotics that are scheduled to be released will be much less effective than those released in the past. For example, when penicillin was first released, it killed 100 percent of some bacteria, such as pneumococcus. No known drug is 100 percent effective any longer.

THE SOLUTION

There is a guardian that can help lower your cholesterol, fight cancer, ward off stomach ulcers, and protect you against food poisoning. It can boost your immune function by producing its own antibiotics, and it is armed with other weapons that are effective against many harmful bacteria, viruses, and fungi. One of its duties is to monitor and control the growth of potentially harmful microorganisms in your body, such as *Candida albicans*. It can also can help cancel out the effects of toxins and environmental pollutants that you can't avoid.

This guardian can prevent and correct many bowel problems,

including constipation, diarrhea, colitis, and irritable bowel syndrome, as well as protect you against urinary tract infections. It also works against migraine headaches, rheumatic and arthritic complaints, and some skin conditions, including acne, psoriasis, and eczema. This guardian also participates in the digestive process, manufactures some important B vitamins, and produces the enzymes you need to digest milk-based foods that provide calcium for strong bones and teeth.

The good news is that you have (or should have) billions of these guardians inside your body right now; they are the friendly bacteria that live and work in your gastrointestinal tract. They build colonies in your small and large intestines and constitute your first line of defense against illness and disease. The health of these friendly bacteria depends on you. What you do that helps—or harms—them ultimately helps or harms your body. Good health begins in your intestinal tract.

HEALTH BEGINS WITHIN

The human body is a complex piece of engineering. Many of its systems are self-policing, including your gastrointestinal tract. Your body works hard to keep you healthy. Your immune system does not shoulder full responsibility for your state of health; its function is to take care of any "bad guys" that escape the attention of the friendly bacteria of your intestinal tract. Even before you realize you are not feeling well, these friendly bacteria are on the job.

The bacteria called *Lactobacillus acidophilus* guard your small intestine, while *Bifidobacteria* protect your large intestine. *Lactobacillus bulgaricus* (the bacteria found in yogurt) is a traveling transient bacteria that aids the other two as it passes through your body. These three major guardians live and work inside your intestinal tract.

It is my hope that by the twenty-first century everyone will be as well-acquainted with friendly bacteria as they are with vitamins. Although scientists have known for a very long time just how important these bacteria really are, the information is only now beginning to make a real impact in the field of medicine overall. Once you discover the facts, which are put before you in this book, you will realize that friendly bacteria are the best friends you have.

It is important to remember that antibiotics are engineered to kill bacteria. However, these drugs cannot tell the difference between the friendly bacteria that are essential to your health and the dangerous bacteria that cause illness and disease. Because so many bad bacteria have evolved into drug-resistant forms, friendly colonies often suffer the most casualties. When you lose too many members of these friendly colonies, your first line of defense is weakened, leaving your body open to infection and disease.

This book will explain how the probiotic (pro-life) organisms that belong in your intestinal tract protect you against many illnesses. The information found within the pages of this book is the result of more than twenty-five years of research and study. It shows you how to get healthy and stay that way by insuring the health of the probiotic guardians that stand between you and disease. You will learn the easy way to make sure that your friendly colonies of probiotic bacteria remain strong.

Part One

Probiotics In Your Life

*R*esidential bacteria form colonies in your gastrointestinal tract, mouth, and vaginal tract. Transient bacteria are travelers that are just passing through. Friendly bacteria—including *Lactobacillus acidophilus, Bifido-bacterium bifidum*, and *Lactobacillus bulgaricus*—are your body's first line of defense against the potentially harmful microorganisms that you inhale or ingest. Probiotics is another term for these friendly bacteria that live and work in your gastrointestinal tract every day of your life. Think of them as the "home guard," a mighty bacterial army that defends your body against dangerous invaders. Having sufficient numbers of these friendly bacteria in residence can help prevent a wide range of health problems.

Part One begins with an introduction to the different types of beneficial bacteria, followed by a brief look at the cultured milk products from ancient times to the present. It includes a look at my life and explains how my family's 700-year history of making yogurt led me to make probiotics my life's work. The structure and function of the gastrointestinal tract are discussed, with an explanation of how the friendly bacteria aid in each stage of digestion.

Part One also includes information on the tremendous impact that friendly bacteria and diet have on good health. Because friendly bacteria are as necessary for babies as they are for adults, a chapter covering the specific use of probiotics for infants and young children is also included. Succeeding chapters cover relevant information on the antibiotic action, antiviral activity, and anti-cancer capabilities of friendly bacteria. Finally, Part One concludes with a chapter on the importance of choosing the right probiotics.

1

Yogurt—Yesterday and Today

*T*he health benefits of friendly bacteria first came to the attention of the general public in 1908, when Dr. Elie Metchnikoff, a Russian biologist, wrote *The Prolongation of Life*. Based on the research that earned him one of the world's top honors, this book stunned the medical and scientific communities. In it, Dr. Metchnikoff recognized that certain white blood cells known as phagocytes ingest and destroy dangerous bacteria, a fact we now know to be true. Dr. Metchnikoff shared the 1908 Nobel Prize in Physiology and Medicine for identifying the process of phagocytosis, an important function of the immune system.

Concurrent with his work on the immune system, and perhaps closer to his heart, Dr. Metchnikoff devoted the last ten years of his life to the study of lactic acid-producing bacteria as a means of increasing life span. After much research, he was convinced that he had discovered why so many Bulgarians lived noticeably longer than other people. This phenomenon, he theorized, was due to their consumption of large quantities of cultured foods, especially yogurt, which he believed help maintain the benign ("friendly") bacteria that live in the gastrointestinal tract. Today, we know his belief to be true.

Dr. Metchnikoff was among the first to recognize the relationship between disease and what he called the "poisons" produced in the bowel. He demonstrated how friendly living bacteria normalize bowel habits and fight disease-carrying bacteria, thereby extending the normal life span. His book persuaded many that living longer is the happy result of an intestinal tract that maintains a healthy daily supply of the cultured bacteria found in yogurt. It was Dr. Metchnikoff who named the primary yogurt-culturing bacteria *Lactobacillus bulgaricus*, in honor of the yogurt-loving Bulgarians.

YOGURT YESTERDAY

The origin of fermented foods and cultured milk products goes so far back that it predates recorded history. Most cultured foods start with milk, which people have been drinking since the dawn of time. The first evidence of the domestication of cows occurred in 9,000 BC in Libya, and while there are no written records that prove these ancient people ate yogurt, the probability is high that they consumed cultured milk products of some sort. India's Ayurvedic writings, dating back to 6,000 BC, indicate that regular consumption of dairy products led to a long and healthy life. In India, the milk of almost every animal, from camels to yaks, continues to be made into cultured foods, including yogurt and cheese, of which there are more than 700 varieties.

Authorities believe that cultured foods first occurred naturally, probably from organisms present in the food itself or in the environment. Because these foods were pleasant tasting, it is likely that people soon learned to save a "starter culture" from a particularly good batch of yogurt or other cultured food. This starter was added to a bowl of fresh milk to induce fermentation.

Most authorities agree that the ancient people of the Middle East ate yogurt regularly. Written records confirm that the conquering armies of Genghis Khan lived on this food. History tells us that by the year 1206, Genghis Khan had conquered all of Mongolia and united the warring tribes under his banner. By 1215, the Mongols held most of the Ch'in Empire and had vanquished Turkistan and Afghanistan. They even penetrated southeastern Europe.

Highly mobile, the Mongols rode small, swift horses that were bred to traverse the vast plains of the Mongolian empire. Every Mongol's wealth was measured by the number of horses he owned, and each soldier traveled with a large string of them. These hardy horses were what helped make this army invincible. Not only did they carry soldiers into battle, they also provided the rich milk that was fermented and enjoyed by every member of the conquering hordes—from the Great Khan to the lowliest slave. Known as kumiss, this is one of the earliest known fermented milk products. Highly nutritious, kumiss not only not sustained the Mongols, it kept them healthy.

Kefir, another cultured milk product, originated in the Caucasus mountains of Russia. It is variously cultured from the milk of goats, sheep, or cows. Its name translates loosely to "pleasure" or "good feeling." Due to its health-promoting properties, kefir was once considered a gift from the gods. Ever since the eighteenth century, kefir has been credited with healing powers. As early travelers to the Caucasus region came home with stories of its powerful healing properties, everyone wanted some of this medicinal miracle food. However, the necessary starter cultures, which were passed from generation to generation among the Moslem tribesmen of the Caucasus, were considered a very real source of family and tribal wealth. The tribes guarded the secret process jealously and protected it with their very lives.

In the early 1900s, the All-Russian Physicians' Society contacted the Blandovs, two brothers who owned cheese factories in the northern Caucasus mountains. The Society asked the brothers for help in obtaining some kefir culture. The brothers put their heads together and came up with a daring idea. Their plan depended on the cooperation of a beautiful young woman named Irina Sakharova, who worked in one of Nicolai Blandov's plants. She was sent to coax a Caucasus prince named Bek-Mirza Barchorov into giving her some culture grains. Although the prince was dazzled by the lovely Irina, he refused to give her any of the precious substance.

The prince made it clear that he wasn't willing to give up the secret of kefir. But he wasn't willing to give up Irina either, and she was kidnapped by the prince's men as she was returning home. Forcibly, they brought her back to the court, where the prince, hoping to win her love, proposed marriage. Irina refused. Eventually, Irina was rescued by the Blandovs. Then, backed by the brothers, she brought her grievance against the prince to the Czar's court. The prince offered Irina gold and jewels as reparation for the wrongs done to her, but she refused. As a settlement of her suit against Prince Bek-Mirza Barchorov, Irina demanded—and got—grains of the precious kefir culture.

In September 1908, Irina Sakharova brought the first bottles of cultured kefir to Moscow, where it was used medicinally with great success. In 1973, Irina, at age 85, received a letter from the Minister of the Food Industry of the USSR. In it, he gratefully acknowledged her primary role in bringing kefir to the Russian people.

My Story
From Yogurt to Probiotics

My family's involvement with cultured milk products can be traced over seven centuries. Yogurt is the ancient "grandmother" of all probiotics, and I was born into a family that was famous for producing the most delicious yogurt of all. By the time I was born, the original culture was centuries old. As a child, I grew up hearing stories about my ancestors and their prosperous yogurt business.

By the beginning of the Second World War, my family had enjoyed great wealth and prosperity for many years. Our yogurt was famous—so famous that we supplied it to the royal family of Yugoslavia. Our appointment as yogurt supplier to the royal court continued until the Axis powers brought down the monarchy in 1941. The royal family fled to England and set up a government in exile, but they never regained the throne.

With the Axis takeover and the rise of Marshal Tito to power, the Yugoslavian government became oppressive. Because of our long loyalty to the royal family and our outspoken opposition to the new government, my family suffered many indignities. Our business and much of our wealth was lost. In October of 1954, my parents and I fled to Vienna, where we immediately applied to the American Embassy for permission to immigrate to the United States.

It was over a year before we received permission to enter the United States. We left Vienna in 1955 and settled in Milwaukee with my mother's brother. Although my uncle was very kind and Milwaukee was a nice place, my father felt suitable business opportunities were lacking, so we left Milwaukee nine months later.

Father decided that California, with its legendary healthy lifestyle, was the land of opportunity he was seeking. In the fall of 1956, we arrived in Hollywood with one hundred dollars and no job prospects. In the early 1960s, my father went into the yogurt business with a goal of producing the best yogurt in America. In order to realize his dream, Father knew he needed a starter culture from our famous family yogurt. He contacted a friend in Yugoslavia, bought him an airline ticket, and had him carry the culture to the United States. Father rented a small ice cream plant in Glendale, California, and named the fledgling company Continental Culture Specialists. He sold liquid yogurt by the gallon and solid yogurt in pint jars. At that time, all yogurt was unflavored.

In September 1966, I started college at UCLA, where I met my husband-to-be, Yordan Trenev. We were married on September 5, 1970. By then I had received my degree and joined the family business full-time. I helped develop our Royal Yogurt line of honey-sweetened and fruit-flavored yogurts. Everybody loved them, including the British royal family, and we sent regular shipments to Buckingham Palace. It pleases me very much that our family yogurt continues to be enjoyed by the crowned heads of Europe.

Back then, we sold our yogurt to health food stores, not supermarkets. Yogurt, however, must be refrigerated, and in the early 1970s, most health food stores didn't have refrigerators. I convinced a number of store owners into literally bringing in their old refrigerators from home to insure proper storage of our fresh yogurt. I also arranged to have our Royal Yogurt delivered along with Hansen's fresh-squeezed juices; this cut delivery costs for both companies.

Around this time, I initiated the shipment of dairy products across state lines. Each state has its own standards governing fresh dairy products, which is why these products are usually "home grown." Even though brand names may be recognized nationally, most dairy product producers have local plants. We needed to service our distributors in Pennsylvania and Florida, which prompted me to make a deal with United Airlines. The airline supplied us with shipping containers into which we packed our fresh yogurt along with dry ice. After successfully transporting the product to Pennsylvania and Florida, we began shipping our yogurt all over the United States. Prior to this, the only perishable items shipped by air across state lines were lobsters and orchids. Now, cold-pack shipping of a number of perishable items is common.

Satisfied with my work at Continental Culture Specialists, I left the company in 1974 to explore new challenges. After studying the science behind cultured products, the commercial end of the yogurt business was no longer enough for me. I wanted to get involved with high-tech research into the health benefits of probiotic cultures, and I began by *acting as a consultant to companies involved in yogurt production. At the same time, I continued studying microbiological research papers and scientific literature on the value of cultured milk products.*

In 1980, I made arrangements with a research facility that gave me access to a laboratory where I began culturing my own probiotic supplements. I processed cultures, supervised the freeze-drying and powdering processes, and even helped with the bottling. Everything was billed and shipped from my home. My husband trucked in dry ice every day to keep the live supplements from deteriorating in the garage, where we were forced to keep them stored.

For many years, I found myself continually frustrated by the lack of established standards for probiotics. Probiotics of the finest quality once competed in the marketplace with products of such poor quality that I knew the consumer could not possibly benefit from them. Without reliable standards in place, there was no way for a consumer to compare the worth of any probiotic products. For example, the benefits of L. acidophilus were quite well-known by then, but even a knowledgeable consumer found it difficult to understand the benefits of a super strain of L. acidophilus compared with the generic supplements (some filled with questionable organisms that contained no acidophilus) that also lined store shelves.

I began working with the Natural Nutritional Foods Association (NNFA) to set standards for probiotic supplements. In 1989, the Association wrote and adopted the NNFA Probiotic Labeling Standard. This ruling requires that probiotic supplement labels list the quantity and identity of the living bacteria present, a viable cell count, an expiration date, certification of the absence of pathogens, storage requirements, and a list of any additional ingredients. Unfortunately, at the time of this writing, virtually none of the probiotic suppliers adheres to these standards.

In 1993, I was honored to be recognized as an authority in the field of probiotic cultures. At the request of the World Health Organization, I was invited to speak on probiotic bacteria at the Fifteenth International Congress of Nutrition in Australia. My audience consisted mainly of scientists and Ph.D.s, and although scientific and medical professionals aren't known for embracing any remedy that isn't drug-oriented, I received a standing ovation.

> *Of course, I was flattered by the enthusiastic response I received, but that really wasn't the important issue. What was important is that the applause from the audience indicated that the medical profession is finally beginning to acknowledge the science supporting the daily use of probiotics. Probioticists aren't relegated to research labs any longer. However, until beneficial bacterial supplements are as well-known as vitamins—and that day is coming—this news remains insider information.*

YOGURT TODAY

Today, yogurt is enjoyed just about everywhere. With the exception of the Chinese, who prefer fermented soy products, milk-cultured yogurt is enjoyed worldwide.

In the 1970s, yogurt consumption rose in the United States by 500 percent. By the mid-1980s, Americans were spending close to $1 billion on yogurt every year. And for the fiscal year ending November 1995, the National Yogurt Association estimated yogurt sales in this country alone at around $1.38 billion.

Yogurt is as familiar as milk in the dairy cases of supermarkets everywhere. It is available fresh or frozen and in regular, low-fat, and nonfat varieties. And talk about flavors—you can now select from a bewildering array of flavors that were unthinkable not so long ago. Most people view yogurt as a wholesome, high-protein, healthy food. It is, and it isn't. It all depends on how the yogurt is made.

The friendly bacteria used to culture true yogurt are *Lactobacillus bulgaricus* and *Streptococcus thermophilus*. When these bacteria are added to milk and allowed to ferment, the resulting culture is a naturally sweet, mildly tangy, smooth, fresh-tasting custard-like treat. And, thanks to the action of the bacteria, true yogurt is almost a "predigested" food. Within an hour after eating yogurt, 90 percent of it is digested. Compare this to a glass of milk, of which only 30 percent is digested in the same amount of time. More importantly, the friendly live bacteria present in true yogurt offer health benefits, some of which are discussed in this book's Preface. More benefits will be discussed in succeeding chapters.

Unfortunately, those colorful little cups of stuff in the supermarket don't qualify as true yogurt. You should be aware that the commercial production of yogurt isn't regulated. There are some loose guidelines that give a list of bacteria that are acceptable as starter organisms, but the bacteria are not ranked according to their health-promoting benefits. Many organisms will cause fermentation, but only living specific strains of L. *bulgaricus* and S. *thermophilus* provide proven health benefits. Often, the least expensive organisms are the most popular with profit-oriented producers.

Although it is frowned upon, some manufacturers still pasteurize their products after the culturing process is complete. This destroys any harmful bacteria lurking in the yogurt; however, it also kills the microorganisms used to cause the fermentation. Therefore, even if the very best bacteria have been used as culturing organisms, they will be destroyed in the pasteurization process. Only living bacteria provide proven health benefits.

If you are like most people, you probably like the sweet fruit-flavored yogurts best. They are the bestsellers. But if you think the addition of fruit adds to the healthy qualities of yogurt, you're mistaken, for several reasons.

First, the fruit that is added to most commercial yogurt is processed, not fresh. Second, the live bacteria used as a culturing agent like the sugars in fruit as much as you do; in fact, they would much rather nibble on the fruit sugar than ferment the milk. Whether the fruit is layered on the top or the bottom, or swirled throughout the yogurt, chemical additives are placed between the fruit and the cultured milk to keep the live bacteria from coming into contact with the fruit.

The manufacturer of one very popular, fruit-flavored yogurt uses a culture called *pima*, which is not a lactobacillus (milk-based) culturing agent at all. What pima produces is slime. This allows the manufacturer to skip adding a thickener to the yogurt. The end result of the pima culture is a homogenous slimy mass that does not separate. If it was sold as plain yogurt, you'd probably spit it out. To hide the slimy texture and odd taste, the manufacturer adds a lot of processed fruit and sugar.

Unfortunately, for all of these reasons, I can't recommend any of the commercially produced yogurts on the market today. I urge you to read labels carefully and try to make an informed choice. It's a shame that this simple, nutrient-rich, health-promoting food has been so commercialized.

Some health food stores promote their own brand of yogurt. Unfortunately, even yogurt sold as "old fashioned" or "homemade" may not have the quality you're looking for. This is because even your health food store suppliers shop for starter cultures in the same places commercial producers shop. It's easier and less expensive to use a manipulated bacteria that has been designed to shorten production time, rather than use truly beneficial strains of *L. bulgaricus* and *S. thermophilus* cultures. The milk will still sour, and the end result will look right and taste right, but, without the right starter culture, the healthy benefits you're looking for will be missing.

If you won't settle for less than the best yogurt, make your own using a starter of *L. bulgaricus* and *S. thermophilus*, which is sold in most health food stores. You'll be surprised at how easy it is. True homemade yogurt is smooth and creamy, faintly sweet, and mildly tangy with a refreshing aftertaste. I promise you, one taste of your own homemade yogurt will convince you it is well worth the very small effort.

If you like yogurt that is sweet and fruity, add your own fresh fruit. If you like it crunchy, add some low-fat, no-sugar-added granola cereal. Health food stores offer a variety of healthy, whole grain cereals that make perfect toppings for a morning bowl of true yogurt.

It seems that everyone is aware of the importance of a well-functioning immune system, but few people give much thought to their digestive processes. Nonetheless, it is well-known that what you eat has a major effect on your health. What you might not know is that your gastrointestinal tract is actually your first line of defense against disease. In the next chapter, you'll understand why.

2

Your Gastrointestinal Tract

Your gastrointestinal tract is a long passageway that begins at your mouth and ends at your anus. It is both a food processor and a fueling station. Fuel equals energy, and this is where the energy to run your body comes from. Nutrients are processed here and passed on to fuel your cells. Your gastrointestinal tract also functions as a trash compactor and waste disposal system. After the nutrients are extracted from food and the water is reabsorbed, the compacted mass of "trash" leaves the body as feces. In addition to these important duties, this is also where the friendly bacteria—your first line of defense—live and work. You should know what goes on in your gastrointestinal tract and just why it is so important to your health and longevity.

The full length of the human digestive tract, from entrance to exit, is five to six times the height of the individual. Using five-and-a-half times as the norm, this means that the digestive system of a three-foot-tall toddler is around sixteen-and-a-half feet, and the gastrointestinal tract of a six-foot-tall adult is thirty-three feet long. It's hard to believe that almost all of that "tubing" is tucked inside your abdomen, but it is.

When you take a bite of food, the route that the food travels from your mouth into your throat, through your esophagus, and into your stomach is a straight highway, but there are many curves ahead. Your small intestine curves around and doubles back on itself several times before it passes material into your large intestine. Your large intestine then goes up your right side, passes under your stomach and pancreas, and comes back down on your left side where it meets the rectum and anus.

YOUR MOUTH AND ESOPHAGUS

Before you take the first bite of food, your "food processor" is ready for action. Digestion begins in your mouth, where the sight and smell of food causes your salivary glands to begin producing digestive enzymes. It is this enzyme-filled saliva that starts the chemical breakdown of food into the simple, basic nutrients your body can use. Once you swallow, food travels through your esophagus, which is about ten inches long in the average adult, and passes into your stomach. This takes only around ten seconds.

YOUR STOMACH

If you were able to open your stomach up fully, and then carefully smooth out all the billions of tiny wrinkles in its lining, its surface area would actually cover a tennis court! Compare your stomach to an elastic bag. After a big Thanksgiving dinner, for example, it can stretch to hold two-and-a-half pints of food. The next time you're cleaning berries in your colander, take a look at just how much space two-and-a-half pints takes up. It's not a good idea to force your stomach to stretch to accept this much food very often, because it puts a strain on your digestive system.

Even before you swallow, digestive juices fill your stomach as it readies itself to accept the coming food. When the food reaches your stomach, the stomach muscles begin to expand and contract, churning the food and mixing it well with digestive juices. Food remains in your stomach from two to four hours while this process takes place. Glands in the stomach wall release digestive enzymes and hydrochloric acid. This specialized acid not only assists in the digestive process, it also helps kill off most unhealthy bacteria.

Other stomach glands produce mucus to protect your stomach wall from being burned by the acidic digestive juices. It was once thought that too much acid caused the holes in the stomach wall known as ulcers. Today, we know that most ulcers are caused by *Helicobacter pylori*, a bacteria that burrows into the stomach lining, causing inflammation in that area. Fortunately, your friendly bacteria can protect you from *H. pylori* and other bad bacteria. You'll see how in Chapter 3.

YOUR SMALL INTESTINE

You might be surprised to know that most of the work of the digestive tract does not take place in the stomach, but in the small intestine. In the average adult, this section of tubing is about twenty-one feet long. It is divided into three areas that join one another—the duodenum, the jejunum, and the ileum.

The walls of the small intestine are not smooth. Despite the length of this part of the gastrointestinal tract, a smooth surface would not provide enough surface area to complete digestion. Millions of tiny hairlike filaments called villi line the intestinal walls. These miniature projections wave back and forth like plants in an aquarium, capturing nutrients from the food as it passes through the small intestine.

Each villus has its own network of capillaries, the tiniest of blood vessels. Amino acids and simple sugars pass through the walls of the villi and into the capillaries, finally entering the bloodstream. The villi also have a vessel connected to the lymphatic system, which is yet another transportation system for liquids. Even when completely broken down, fat molecules are too large to travel through the tiny capillaries, so they travel through lymph vessels instead.

The Duodenum

At the upper end of the small intestine, a C-shaped section called the duodenum receives digestive juices directly from the pancreas, liver, and gallbladder. Without the help provided by these glands, the digestive process would fail.

The Pancreas

The pancreas secretes both digestive juices and the hormones insulin and glucagon. Coupled with hormones from other endocrine glands, the pancreatic hormones play a primary role in the regulation of carbohydrate metabolism. When the pancreas secretes insufficient insulin, the result is diabetes mellitus. When it puts out too much insulin, the result is hypoglycemia, or low blood sugar.

Every day, the pancreas secretes up to two pints of enzyme-rich digestive juices into the duodenum. These juices are important for the digestion of all types of food, especially carbohydrates. The pancreatic juices continue the breakdown of carbohydrates into sugars that started in the mouth. The liver then converts these sugars into glucose, the blood sugar used by the body for energy. Other pancreatic enzymes continue working on the breakdown of proteins and fats that began in the stomach.

The Liver

The liver is your largest internal organ, weighing between three and four pounds in the average adult. The liver receives its blood supply from two sources, the heart and the small intestine. The heart provides approximately one-fifth of this blood, which is oxygenated, while the remaining nutrient-rich blood comes from the pancreas.

A major part of the digestive system, the liver plays other important roles as well. For example, it breaks down old red blood cells and processes potential poisons for removal from the body. These poisons include nicotine and alcohol, which the liver can process in small amounts, and drugs that have served their purpose. It also detoxifies certain harmful substances produced in the intestines, such as phenols and ammonia, which it turns into urea, a compound found in urine.

Another vital function performed by the liver is storage. Carbohydrates in the form of glycogen remain in the liver until energy is called for by the brain, muscles, and organs; then the glycogen is converted into glucose and transported to where it is needed. This function is especially important to your brain, since it cannot store glucose. In order for you to think properly, your brain depends on the steady supply of glucose energy that your liver provides. The liver also processes proteins, vitamins, and many other compounds used by your body.

To do its part in the digestive process, the liver produces a thick, greenish fluid called bile, which makes the digestion of fats possible by making them water-soluble. Bile is stored in the gallbladder until needed. When you eat a fat-laden meal, your liver prepares for the onslaught by filling the gallbladder with extra bile.

The Jejunum and Ileum

Once the important work by the pancreas and liver is complete, the partially digested food passes from the duodenum to the other two sections of the small intestine. The middle section is called the jejunum, and the final section is called the ileum. These areas of the small intestine also produce digestive juices. Millions of glands in their walls secrete about five pints of enzyme-rich juices every day.

PROCESSING FOODS AND LIQUIDS

When the food you have eaten has finally been broken down into its basic components—amino acids and simple sugars—the molecules are small enough to be absorbed into the bloodstream for transport where they are needed. The average adult absorbs about ten quarts of processed food and liquids every day.

Processing Carbohydrates

Vegetables, fruits, and grains supply your body with carbohydrates, starches, and sugars. Carbohydrates are the easiest foods for your body to digest. Many experts believe that about 60 percent of your total calorie intake should come from carbohydrate-rich foods, such as whole fruits, vegetables, and grains. As soon as you begin chewing, carbohydrates begin to break down into glucose, the simple sugar that is used by your body for energy. If you chew something salty long enough, it will begin to taste sweet—a direct result of the enzymes in your saliva at work.

After the breakdown of carbohydrates into glucose by your small intestine, the glucose passes into your bloodstream, which carries it to other parts of your body. Any of your 75 trillion cells can use it right away for energy, while some of it is stored as glycogen in your liver and muscles until it is needed.

Processing Protein

During the digestive process, proteins are broken down into subunits called amino acids. Your body requires approximately twenty-two amino acids in a specific pattern to make human protein. Fourteen of these acids can be produced by an adult body. The remaining eight, called essential amino acids, must be supplied to the body daily. To find out how many grams of complete protein you must eat every day to furnish your body with sufficient amino acids, divide your body weight by two. For example, someone who weighs 140 pounds needs seventy grams of high-quality protein every day.

The proteins found in meat, fish, eggs, whole grains, and beans supply your body with amino acids. The breakdown of proteins into chains of amino acids begins in the stomach, but occurs mostly in the small intestine. Once this breakdown is complete, your bloodstream carries the amino acids to where they are needed.

Amino acids are the raw materials your body uses, first, to manufacture red blood cells (hemoglobin) and, second, to make blood plasma proteins. Once these important requirements are met, they are used to build new cells and tissues, such as skin, and to repair and maintain old cells. Proteins are especially important while the body is growing, but adults still require them every day to repair cells and tissues.

Processing Fats

Dairy products (not including nonfat items), eggs, meats, and oils supply your body with fats. It takes your body longer to break down fats than any other food. This breakdown process begins in the stomach and is completed in the small intestine. Fats move to other parts of the body through the lymphatic system.

Some dietary fat is essential to good health—although not as much as many people consume. Fats carry fat-soluble vitamins to your cells, and surround and cushion your internal organs. Fat is also used for energy storage. Extra fat is stored in your liver or under your skin. Anyone struggling with a weight problem is aware of this type of fat storage.

The average American consumes 40 percent of his or her daily calories from fat in a typical day. The American Heart Association suggests no more than 30 percent of one's daily calories come from fat, with 25 percent being even better.

With the amount of daily fat you eat based on caloric intake, you must first establish how many calories you need in a day. In order for the average adult to maintain his or her weight, he or she must consume about 15 calories for each pound they weigh. Let's say you weigh 130 pounds. To maintain this weight, you would need to consume about 1,950 calories a day:

$$
\begin{array}{rl}
130 & \text{pounds} \\
\times\ \ 15 & \text{calories} \\
\hline
1{,}950 & \text{total daily calories}
\end{array}
$$

Next, multiply the total calories by 0.25 (25 percent) to determine the maximum number of calories that should come from fat:

$$
\begin{array}{rl}
1{,}950 & \text{total daily calories} \\
\underline{\times\ 0.25} & \text{percent} \\
487 & \text{total calories from fat}
\end{array}
$$

Finally, as 1 gram of fat has 9 calories, divide the total calories by 9 to determine the total daily fat-gram allowance:

$$
\begin{array}{rl}
487 & \text{total calories from fat} \\
\underline{\div\ 9} & \text{calories per fat gram} \\
54 & \text{total daily fat grams}
\end{array}
$$

At first, 54 grams of fat may seem like a great deal, but consider that one tablespoon of butter (or margarine) spread on your morning toast contains fourteen grams. You can see how easy it is for those fat grams to accumulate. And watch out for processed foods. They are characteristically high in both calories and fat content.

If you're monitoring your cholesterol intake, limit your consumption of animal fat to 2,000 milligrams daily. This amount is generally considered safe on a low-cholesterol diet.

Vitamins and Minerals

Vitamins and minerals—important for healthy body functioning—pass unchanged from the small intestine into the bloodstream or lymphatic ducts. Evidence shows the bioavailability of calcium, zinc, iron, manganese, copper, and phosphorus is increased in yogurt when compared to milk. This is due to the production of lactic acid, which allows for better absorption of minerals in the instestines. Other studies suggest vitamin production by lactobacilli and bifidobacteria, and better bioavailability of these vitamins due to acidification of the small and large intestines.

THE LARGE INTESTINE

The large intestine is your waste disposal system. Once all the useful components of food have been absorbed, the indigestible parts are sent to the large intestine for final disposal.

Humans cannot digest cellulose, the fibrous carbohydrate present in plant foods. This dietary fiber, also known as roughage, aids in the waste removal process and helps prevent constipation. Good sources of fiber include vegetables, fruits, and whole grains.

The indigestible parts of food move from the small intestine into the large intestine, where water and needed chemicals are absorbed back into the bloodstream and recycled. The remaining material travels on to the rectum and passes out of the body as waste.

Like the small intestine, the large intestine is also divided into three sections—the ascending colon, the transverse colon, and the descending colon. The ascending colon receives processed food from the small intestine through a connection on the right side. It then turns and ascends upward. When it almost reaches the waist, it becomes the transverse colon, which dips down under the pancreas and stomach, turns back up slightly, and then crosses over to the left side. The descending colon travels down the left side, turns inward, and extends to the midpoint of the body, where it meets the rectum and anus. It can take anywhere from eighteen to sixty-eight hours, or even longer, for food residue to pass through the entire large intestine.

FOOD FOR THOUGHT

Every system of your body is vitally important to your health, but you have more control over your digestive system than you do over any other.

Your heart beats and your lungs take in and expel air throughout your lifetime. These systems are termed autonomic (think automatic) systems because they are programmed to run automatically. Of course, how well your cardiovascular and respiratory systems function does depend in large part on your lifestyle choices, but you don't have to make a conscious effort to start your heart every morning when you wake up, and you don't have to remember to breathe.

Your gastrointestinal tract is different. Once you swallow a bite of food, your body takes over the digestive process and runs automatically. With the exception of dangerous microbes that you can't avoid, what you put in your mouth is under your personal control.

Your body is composed of about 75 trillion cells. Every cell—from the largest four-foot-long nerve cell to the smallest sperm cell—requires nutrients to provide the fuel it needs to do its work. Each cell is fueled by the nutrients present in the food you eat; they are dependent on you for the materials they need to build, repair, maintain, and control every system in your body.

In 1987, the USDA funded a study to find out if the average American was eating a diet that provided ten essential nutrients. Out of the 21,000 people who participated in the study, not one was taking in the Recommended Daily Allowance (RDA) of the ten targeted nutrients considered essential for good health.

CONCLUSION

How well you feed your cells plays a large part in determining how healthy you are and how long you will live. Think about this: by the time you are presented with a birthday cake that has seventy blazing candles, your body will have processed between 60,000 and 100,000 pounds of food. That's 30,000 to 50,000 tons!

In the next chapter, you will meet the friendly bacteria that live in your gastrointestinal tract and aid in the digestive process. Feeding your cells well is vitally important, but, without the help of these front-line guardians, all sorts of problems can beset the human body. Once you have learned the rest of the story, you'll understand exactly why I say that your health begins in your gastrointestinal tract.

3

Your First Line of Defense

*O*ver time, human beings have developed a symbiotic relationship with beneficial bacteria. The immune system swings into action at the first sign that any dangerous microbe has escaped the lethal attentions of the defenders of the gastrointestinal tract, yet the beneficial bacteria are never attacked. The body somehow realizes that these friendly bacteria are essential to health, and leaves them alone. Indeed, I suspect the immune system welcomes their help.

Your gastrointestinal tract is where it all begins. This is where the war between the good guys and the bad guys can be won quickly, but it's also where crucial battles may be lost. When colonies of beneficial bacteria are present in sufficient numbers, chances are you won't even know you're under siege. However, if you have a deficiency of friendly bacteria and have lost too many colonists—for whatever reason—you will fall ill very quickly when an alien bacteria invades your body.

Around one-third of the dry weight of fecal material consists of both live and dead bacteria. A thorough analysis of one small sample of human feces could take over a year to complete. That is why, when a laboratory is asked to analyze a stool sample, they are given a short list of organisms that your doctor believes may be making you sick. In the case of suspected food poisoning, for example, the lab may be required to test only for *E. coli* and *Salmonella* bacteria, two of the most common culprits present in the food chain.

COMMON INHABITANTS OF
THE GASTROINTESTINAL TRACT

Over 400 species of bacteria inhabit your digestive tract, with different species occupying other regions of your body. The thousands of billions of tiny bacteria living in the average adult's gastrointestinal tract weigh about three-and-a-half pounds. You actually have more bacterial cells in your intestines than the total number of cells in your body. Here is a brief look at some of the common microscopic organisms that "reside" in the different areas of the gastrointestinal tract.

In the Mouth

Gateway to the body, your mouth contains a large number of bacteria that thrive in saliva. In addition to the important digestive enzymes that begin the chemical breakdown of food as you chew, saliva contains between 10,000 and 1 billion microorganisms per milliliter (⅕ teaspoon). Although some bacteria found in the mouth can cause cavities if they are present for too long, most are neutral occupants. In varying numbers, your saliva contains *Streptococci, Lactobacilli, Veillonella, Bacteroides, Staphylococci, and Corynebacteria.* Also present are fusiform bacilli and spirochetes, which can combine to produce fusospirochetal disease—a form of trenchmouth or Vincent's angina—an acute form of gingivitis.

In the Stomach

During the digestive process, the stomach secretes both digestive enzymes and hydrochloric acid. These elements continue the digestive process that began in the mouth. In contrast to the great number of bacteria present in your mouth, your stomach contains only about 1,000 per milliliter. This is because many of the microorganisms you swallow cannot survive the hostile, acidic environment of the stomach. This is very fortunate when you think about the number of unfriendly bacteria that are present in the food chain and water supplies.

The length of time that food remains in your stomach is just one of the factors that helps determine how many and what species of bacteria survive the digestive acids. Several other factors determine how well bacteria, both helpful and harmful, survive in the lower regions of your gastrointestinal tract. These include diet, pH factors, environmental exposures, and proper peristalsis.

Diet

The type of food you eat impacts the bacteria that inhabit your body. For example, a bifidogenic diet, consisting of a high intake of complex carbohydrates, including vegetables, fruits, and grains, encourages high levels of friendly bifidobacteria in your large intestine. On the other hand, a high intake of meats actually fosters a buildup of putrefactive bacteria. This is because meats (and fats) take a long time to break down to become fully digested.

pH Factor

Level of acidity is determined by the environment's pH factor. pH stands for hydrogen potential. A pH level of 7 indicates a neutral environment. Any pH number above 7 signifies an alkaline environment, while numbers below 7 indicate an acidic environment.

The degree of acidity in the gastrointestinal tract contributes to bacterial colonization of some species and helps in the destruction of others. Maintaining the normal acidic environment of your stomach is very important. Be aware that the overuse of antacids, including over-the-counter acid-neutralizing products, prescription drugs, and even that old standby, bicarbonate of soda, upsets the acid balance and allows harmful bacteria to survive in this usually hostile region.

Environmental Exposure

People living in certain areas of the world, such as the tropics, are often exposed to microbial infections. Although Americans were once believed to be relatively safe from infection by harmful microbes, this is no longer true. Both the food chain and many water systems have been infiltrated with dangerous organisms. Unless proper precautions are observed, in all likelihood, your family will be (or has been) exposed to some of them.

Peristaltic Action

Peristalsis is the name given to the wave-like motion caused by muscles when they alternately expand and contract. Peristalsis occurs from the top of your gastrointestinal tract to the bottom; it is what keeps the contents moving along this very long passageway. Poor peristaltic action is often the result of an insufficient amount of fluid and fiber in the diet.

Any bacteria that survive passage through the acidic environment of your stomach, and many do, are passed on to your small intestine. When peristalsis is slowed or interrupted, food becomes stagnant and may putrefy. This stagnant, rotting food becomes fertile ground for the overgrowth of yeast and harmful bacteria. Poor peristalsis may also cause constipation, which can lead to diverticulitis—a condition in which food is trapped in small pouchlike areas of the intestines called diverticula. Once trapped, the diverticula may become inflamed or infected, resulting in pain, fever, and chills.

In the Small Intestine

Your small intestine is not only the area where most food digestion takes place, it is also where any harmful bacteria that have survived their travels through the stomach arrive next. The upper parts of your small intestine—the duodenum and the jejunum—are sparsely populated with only about 10,000 organisms per milliliter of contents. These are mainly the transient (traveling) bacteria that stay in the gastrointestinal tract for a relatively short time.

However, further down in the ileum there is a varied and permanent population of organisms. Here, the population may number between 100,000 and 10 million organisms per milliliter. The types of bacteria found here include *Streptococci;* small amounts of *Bacteroides;* a variety of yeasts and enterobacteria, some of which are harmful; bifidobacteria, a friendly neighbor that lives primarily in the large intestine; and lactobacilli. *Lactobacillus acidophilus* is the most important of the friendly bacteria that live in your small intestines.

The Lactobacillus Family

Lactobacillus acidophilus, L. bulgaricus, and L. casei are all beneficial members of the lactobacillus family. Both *L. bulgaricus* and *L. casei* are transient bacteria, commonly found in varying numbers in the intestines as they pass through. They come from dairy products you eat, including yogurt, milk, and cheese.

All lactobacilli have some common traits. The prefix *lacto*—from the Latin for "milk"—indicates that these bacteria prefer a milk-based growing medium. Another common characteristic they share is the production of the enzyme *lactase,* which is essential for the digestion of milk sugar (*lactose*). They also produce lactic acid from carbohydrates, which creates an acidic environment in the digestive tract that helps get rid of any harmful microorganisms that thrive in an alkaline environment.

Some bacteria can live only in an oxygen-free environment, while others need small amounts of oxygen, just as we do. Because of their ability to grow in both the presence or absence of oxygen, lactobacilli are considered facultative anaerobic bacteria. These varying characteristics are very important to the defenders of your body. For example, by using up all available oxygen in their habitat, the friendly "breathing" bacteria deny oxygen to the harmful species that require it.

By far, the most important bacterial resident of your small intestine is *L. acidophilus.* This is the colonizer, the inhabitant that constitutes your first line of defense against alien invaders, as well as opportunistic organisms like yeasts, which can take over the area and spread throughout your body when the defensive occupying forces are weakened. *L. acidophilus* bacteria even help keep your heart healthy by lowering the levels of cholesterol in your blood—an effect that is explained further in Chapter 4.

When *L. acidophilus* bacteria are present in sufficient numbers, they prevent invading pathogens and opportunistic organisms from finding "parking spaces" along the walls of the intestine, where nutrients cross into the bloodstream. If too many harmful bacteria manage to set up colonies, nutrient absorption can be blocked. Fortunately, when the walls are crowded with acidophilus colonizers, there is no room for newcomers and no way for opportunistic organisms to exceed their boundaries. A very desirable characteristic of some *L. acidophilus* super strains is that they adhere naturally to the walls of your intestines. These strains, known as sticker strains, are the most desirable because they hang onto their parking spaces with great tenacity—without harming the intestinal wall. Most pathogens, like disease-carrying *E. coli,* literally bore holes in the intestinal wall, causing micro-infections.

Although most commercial probiotics don't contain them, certain super strains of beneficial bacteria also act to inhibit undesirable microorganisms by their production of hydrogen peroxide, acids, and natural antibiotics. These substances threaten the existence of harmful bacteria.

Have you ever found yourself in an atmosphere in which you didn't feel comfortable? Instinctively, didn't you want to remove yourself from that environment as soon as possible? The same concept applies to harmful bacteria. Your friendly "good guys" actually create an internal environment that is so hostile to pathogens that these "bad guys" can't wait to vacate the premises. They leave quickly and end up being excreted.

In the Large Intestine

The large intestine is primarily an anaerobic environment—no oxygen is present. This area of your gastrointestinal tract is where the highest concentration of bacteria is found. It houses anywhere from 100 billion to 1,000 billion bacterial microorganisms per milliliter. Remember, a milliliter is only ⅕ of a teaspoon.

By the time the food reaches the large intestine, it is a watery mass and all of its useful nutrients have been absorbed. The primary responsibility of the large intestine is to dispose of this waste, but first it must reclaim or recycle the water, changing the matter into solid material. The waste is then quickly sent on to be expelled from the body.

This recycling process must be performed quickly before the residual matter putrefies and becomes toxic. Another reason for this haste is that many dangerous organisms feed off the putrefying waste. The challenge is to expel the waste before it becomes a nutrient base for harmful bacteria. It is for this reason that chronic constipation can be both uncomfortable and decidedly dangerous.

When resident friendly bacteria are present in sufficient numbers in the large intestine, very little putrefaction occurs and waste matter passes through in a timely fashion. However, numerous problems arise when there aren't enough beneficial bacteria. You usually harbor the same total number of bacteria in your large intestine, but ratios of various groups can shift disastrously. Bad bacteria can multiply and attach themselves to the intestinal walls, crowding out the defenders. Chemicals that are potentially carcinogenic can turn into true cancer-causing agents when harmful bacteria get a toehold in the region. Also, bacterial infections in the intestinal walls, such as ulcerative colitis, become a real possibility when the levels of beneficial bacteria fall.

Bifidobacteria, although present in the lower region of the small intestine are found mostly in the large intestine. They are the region's primary defenders.

Bifidobacteria

The friendly bifidobacteria found in the large intestine include *Bifidobacterium bifidum*, *Bifidobacterium longum*, and *Bifidobacterium infantis*. They are beneficial to babies as well as adults. (Information on the benefits of bifidobacteria on babies is found in Chapter 5.)

As discussed earlier, the lower region of your small intestine is home to small numbers of bifidobacteria, but the largest colonies reside in your large intestine. They are (or should be) the major inhabitants of this area of your gastrointestinal tract.

When bifidobacteria are present in sufficient strength, they compete ferociously for both nutrients and attachment sites along the intestinal walls. Opportunistic organisms—including the yeast fungus *Candida albicans*, and pathogenic invaders that sneak in—are always seeking a chance to colonize and multiply. But they cannot exist without food, and they must have a place to attach themselves. When bifidobacteria colonies are healthy and strong, these "bad guys" are forced to pass through the tract and out of the body.

Another way bifidobacteria protect themselves (and you) is by producing acetic and lactic acids, which create a hostile environment for dangerous microbes that require an alkaline atmosphere. Bifidobacteria also thrive happily without oxygen, so the aerobic bacteria that need to "breathe" cannot survive passage through this area.

Bifidobacteria produce some important B-complex vitamins that you can't live without; they also assist in the dietary management of some liver conditions. In addition, they act against certain harmful bacteria lurking in the region and prevent them from altering nitrates (present in food and water) into nitrites, which are known cancer-causing agents.

WHAT'S IN A NAME?

You've been introduced to your first line of defenders, and you're on a first-name basis with these friendly inhabitants of your gastrointestinal tract. However, before you learn about their scientific documentation of powers, you'll need to become a little better acquainted with them.

When Shakespeare asked, "What's in a name?" he went on to answer, "A rose by any other name would smell as sweet." This may be true of roses, but it does not apply to bacteria. In many cases, a genus or family may contain all good or all bad bacteria, but not always. For example, the genus *Lactobacillus* has no pathogenic species, but some genuses contain bacterial species that go both ways.

When you hear the word *Streptococcus,* you may automatically cringe and think of strep throat. But strep throat comes from *Streptococcus pyogenes,* not from *Streptococcus thermophilus,* which is actually a very friendly transient bacteria common to the human intestines. As you already know, when combined with *L. bulgaricus, S. thermophilus* is half of the duo used to culture yogurt.

In addition, not all friendly bacteria with the same family name have equal powers. Different strains of the friendly intestinal bacteria vary widely in their abilities to protect themselves (and you). Some strains are weak, while others are powerful, but the family resemblance is strong. Microorganisms have three names: genus, species, and strain.

The genus, which is always capitalized, refers primarily to the shape of the organism. This is a broad classification of family members with common distinguishing characteristics. For example, all cats, from the lion on the savanna to the family pet on the sofa, belong to the genus *Felis.* The family resemblance is obvious even to the casual observer. They look alike and, except for size, have the same general shape.

The species classification narrows things further. Different species of the *Felis* family, from tigers to tabbies, are so closely related that it is easy to arrive at the conclusions that all cats eat meat, nurse their babies, and like to sleep in the sun. But knowing this doesn't tell you that tigers are ferocious predators, while the finicky feline who shares your home may turn her nose up at a certain brand of cat food.

The strain is an organism's most specific name. This designation is what separates the men from the boys, so to speak. Some strains of beneficial bacteria have super powers, some are better at certain things than others, and other strains are so weak they have no abilities worth mentioning. For example, all species of the genus *Lactobacillus* are friendly. They can't hurt you, but many of them can't help you either. The strain is an all-important designation.

As people are probably most familiar with *Lactobacillus,* let's use it as an example for describing these classifications. *Lactobacillus* is the genus. Both *acidophilus* and *bulgaricus* are species of *Lactobacillus*. DDS-1 and NAS are two of the many strains of *L. acidophilus*, just as LB-51 and DDS-12 are particular strains of *L. bulgaricus*. All of these strains are designated as "super strains," because they possess the most power and are most active on your behalf. (Detailed information on super strains is presented in Chapter 10.) The following is an abbreviated look at a *Lactobacillus* family tree.

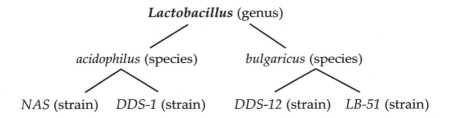

Lactobacillus (genus)

acidophilus (species)   *bulgaricus* (species)

NAS (strain)   *DDS-1* (strain)   *DDS-12* (strain)   *LB-51* (strain)

The friendly bacterial defenders use their weapons against harmful intruders to protect their territory. They also act to control opportunistic organisms, primarily yeasts, and keep them from overstepping their boundaries. Your body is their universe. They know nothing beyond the dark, damp, tubular confines of your gastrointestinal tract, yet the actions they take to protect themselves also protect you.

CONCLUSION

The beneficial bacteria that inhabit your gastrointestinal tract are absolutely essential to your health and well-being. Keeping you healthy isn't solely the responsibility of your immune system. Without strong and viable colonies of both lactobacteria and bifidobacteria, your body will lose the all-important services of these first-line defenders.

The protective powers of beneficial bacteria are many, and will be detailed in subsequent chapters of this book. But before discussing the many ways in which friendly bacteria protect you against illness and disease, let's see just how much they do for you in the realm of nutrition.

4

Your Diet and Friendly Bacteria

You must eat to live. This is a given. However, far too many of us live to eat; that is, we eat things that taste good, not things that necessarily do our bodies good. In this chapter, you'll see how friendly bacteria not only help with your body's nutrient needs, but how they can protect you by lowering your levels of "bad" cholesterol, which can cause atherosclerosis and increase your risk of heart attack.

Eating right means supplying your body with the perfect balance of essential nutrients required to maintain good health. Proper nutrients are needed for normal organ development and functioning, reproduction, growth and maintenance, optimum activity levels and working efficiency, and resistance to infection and disease. Your body also needs essential nutrients to repair bodily damage or injury at the cellular level. It's up to you to supply these nutrients.

GOOD-FOR-YOU FOOD

To qualify as good-for-you food, it should be a source of the nutrients required for good health. This includes foods that supply carbohydrates, essential fatty acids, proteins, vitamins, minerals, enzymes, and trace elements that are in a "bioavailable" form. This means that your body can break down and metabolize the individual nutrients into easily-used, absorbable components. Unless a food is digestible, your body cannot sort out the nutrients, render them available, and then assimilate them.

No single nutrient source—not even real yogurt—can support all of your body's systems. However, the fermentation process carried out by beneficial bacteria greatly enhances the digestibility of cultured foods. In most instances, the nutrients in cultured foods are virtually predigested for you by the fermentation bacteria.

YOGURT AND LACTOSE INTOLERANCE

It is estimated that more than half the people in the world are lactose-intolerant; that is, they are unable to digest lactose (milk sugar). Lactose intolerance is caused by a lack of the digestive enzyme lactase, which converts lactose into a form the body can use, such as glucose or galactose. When a lactose intolerant individual drinks a glass of milk, eats a hot fudge sundae, or ingests any milk product, some or all of the lactose these products contain remains undigested and ferments in the colon. The result is diarrhea, gas, bloating, and abdominal cramps.

The lactase enzyme is commonly missing in those whose ancestors are from southern Europe, Asia, or Africa—countries where milk is not present in the diet once a child is weaned off breast milk. After generations, this lack of milk drinking causes the body to "forget" how to produce the enzyme lactase. Obviously, those who are lactose intolerant must restrict their intake of such foods.

Lactobacilli are known to produce lactase, which helps stimulate the body's own production of lactase. This means that when lactobacilli are present in strong numbers, many people who are lactose intolerant are able to enjoy milk products. Furthermore, studies have demonstrated that people who are lactose-intolerant and unable to drink even nonfat milk can digest yogurt easily. I mean real yogurt, of course, and you must understand the distinction. This benefit is not found in pasteurized yogurt or in any form of yogurt that has no active cultures. The pasteurization of commercial yogurt, after the culturing process is complete, not only destroys some of the nutrients, it kills off most of the friendly bacteria. True yogurt must have active cultures that are able to produce lactase.

However, heat treatment (pasteurization) of milk before yogurt is cultured is necessary to insure vigorous growth of the culture and to get what is considered a "good set." The loss of nutrients that occurs during the pasteurization of milk is more than compensated for by the nutritional benefits of the culturing process.

Those who cannot break down casein, a protein found in milk, must avoid milk and milk products altogether. (For additional information on casein intolerance, see the inset below.)

THE BIOAVAILABILITY OF CALCIUM

Calcium is the most abundant mineral in the body. Your body contains about two-and-a-half pounds of calcium, most of which is in your bones and teeth. Without sufficient calcium, you are at risk of suffering from osteoporosis as you get older. Mainly absorbed through the small intestine, calcium is needed to carry nerve signals, to contract muscles, to clot blood, to help your heart function, and to work with enzymes.

Only about 20 to 30 percent of the calcium you take in every day is absorbed by your body. The rest is eliminated in urine, feces, and sweat. For the average adult, the RDA of calcium is 800 milligrams. As you get older, your calcium requirement increases because the absorption process slows down. Older adults, pregnant women, and nursing mothers need up to 1,200 milligrams of calcium daily. The RDA for growing children is from 800 to 1,200 milligrams.

Clearly, calcium is a very important nutrient. It is present in many foods, but most abundantly in milk products, especially real yogurt. One cup of real yogurt supplies more than half your daily calcium

---

Casein Intolerance

For the same genetic reason some people are lactose intolerant, a small number of people are casein intolerant. Casein is a protein found in milk and milk products. Those who cannot digest casein experience the same symptoms—gas, abdominal cramps, and diarrhea—as those who cannot digest lactose.

While the friendly lactobacilli are able to produce the enzyme lactase, which enables many who are lactose intolerant to partake in varying amounts of milk products, research has not yet shown that the beneficial bacteria can produce the necessary enzyme to break down casein. Unfortunately, those who are casein intolerant must avoid milk products altogether.

requirement. Table 4.1, below, compares the calcium levels found in a number of foods.

In an article entitled, "Nutritive Value of Yogurt," by Dr. J.L. Rasic, published in *The Journal of Cultured Dairy Products*, Dr. Rasic points out that calcium and other minerals are better absorbed from yogurt than from milk. This is because the combination of acid production and improved protein digestibility (courtesy of the friendly culturing bacteria) greatly enhances calcium absorption by improving the bioavailability of the nutrients.

Many authorities argue that taking a calcium supplement is just as good as eating a bowl of yogurt or drinking a glass of milk, but there is another benefit to being able to digest milk products—they are excellent sources of high-quality protein.

THE BIOAVAILABILITY OF PROTEINS

Your body requires a daily supply of proteins. Proteins are necessary for growth, development, and cellular repair. A source of heat and

Table 4.1 Calcium Levels of Foods

FOOD	AMOUNT	CALCIUM CONTENT
Nonfat plain yogurt	8 ounces	425 mg
Lowfat plain yogurt	8 ounces	415 mg
Fresh collard greens, cooked	1 cup	357 mg
Lowfat fruit-flavored yogurt	8 ounces	314–345 mg
Skim milk	8 ounces	302 mg
Whole milk	8 ounces	291 mg
Soft-serve vanilla ice cream (11% fat)	8 ounces	236 mg
Part-skim mozzarella cheese	1 ounce	207 mg
Canned pink salmon	3 ounces	167 mg
Calcium-enriched fruit juices	8 ounces	150–300 mg
Lowfat cottage cheese	8 ounces	156 mg
Fresh broccoli, cooked	1 cup	136 mg

energy, proteins also act in the formation of hormones, enzymes, and antibodies, while maintaining the body's acid-alkaline balance.

To make proteins bioavailable, the body breaks down the large protein molecules into simpler units called amino acids. Twenty-two amino acids in a specific pattern are needed to make human protein— the only kind your body can use. All but eight of these amino acids can be produced in the adult body. The eight that your body cannot make are called *essential* amino acids because they must be supplied in the daily diet. If even one essential amino acid is missing, even temporarily, protein synthesis will drop or stop altogether.

In an adult, protein deficiency results in loss of vigor and stamina, mental depression, profound weakness, poor resistance to infection, impaired healing of wounds, and a slow recovery from illnesses. Even your hair and nails will be affected. The problem is worse for children.

To determine your protein requirements, divide your body weight in half. The result will show how many daily grams of protein you need. For example, a person weighing 180 pounds requires about 90 grams of protein daily, or approximately three ounces (there are slightly more than 30 grams in one ounce).

In order for your body to make use of proteins, they must be broken down into free amino acids or peptides, which are very small amino acid chains. The proteins in natural yogurt, which contains live lactobacteria, arrive with the process of digestion well underway. Even before you take a spoonful, friendly bacteria have begun to convert proteins, fats, and milk sugars into easily-digested components. The nutrients in natural yogurt are immediately bioavailable and ready for use.

In their 1973 paper, "Nutritional and Therapeutic Aspects of Lactobacilli," published in *The Journal of Applied Nutrition*, Drs. K.M. Shahani and B.A. Friend demonstrate that there is up to a 10 percent improvement in the quality of protein found in cultured yogurt as compared to the skim milk from which it was made.

Dr. J.L. Rasic confirmed that yogurt-fed animals have a higher rate of healthy growth than animals who are fed the usual chow. This is one way in which the biological value of a food can be measured. This value is also based on the number of amino acids it contains, especially the essential ones. A food's value is further mitigated by its digestibility and the bioavailability of its amino acids. Table 4.2 lists a

Table 4.2 Biological Values of Protein-Rich Foods

FOOD	BIOLOGICAL VALUE
Yogurt (goat's milk)	90.5 %
Yogurt (sheep's milk)	89.3 %
Yogurt (cow's milk)	87.3 %
Milk, cow's	84.5 %
Fish	76 %
Beef	74.3 %
Chicken	74.3 %
Whole wheat	64.7 %
Corn (maize)	59.4 %

number of protein-rich foods and their biological values as determined by Dr. Rasic. Although we tend to think of meat products as the best protein sources, it is actually dairy foods that provide the most protein, with yogurt at the top of the list. As you can see, the protein and essential amino acids in yogurt made from goat's milk is 90.5 percent available to your body for use.

The fermentation process measurably increases the protein levels of cultured foods. Even protein-rich foods like milk actually contain more protein after fermentation than they do before the friendly bacteria interact with them. For example, when lactobacteria are used to culture cheese-whey into yogurt, there is a net gain of 7 percent in the protein content of the final product. This additional protein is evidence of the friendly bacteria at work.

When you eat a cultured food such as yogurt, you not only receive the bonus of extra protein, but it is delivered in a partially predigested, completely bioavailable form that your body will greatly appreciate. These welcome benefits have also been proven in the Far East, where fermented, protein-rich beans and other vegetables comprise a major element of the diet.

There are, however, substances in beans, for example, that make them difficult for some people to digest. These anti-nutrient chemicals include phytates and trypsin-inhibitors. If you dread serving beans because of their uncomfortable aftereffects, you should know that when certain beans are fermented, such as soybeans that are then transformed into bean curd (tofu), the offending chemicals are mysteriously missing. They are either destroyed by the fermentation process, or the friendly bacteria somehow act to prevent them from affecting the gastrointestinal tract. However it happens, it's a welcome development.

ENHANCING VITAMIN B-COMPLEX PRODUCTION

B-complex vitamins are water-soluble nutrients that can be cultivated from bacteria, yeasts, fungi, or molds. Because they are water-soluble, excess B-complex vitamins are excreted, not stored in the body. For this reason, they must be continually replaced every day. These vitamins are found in such meager amounts in the American diet that most people lack at least some of them.

Many lactobacillus cultures require additional levels of B-complex vitamins in order to grow, so they manufacture them. In his 1983 paper, "Role of Dairy Foods Containing Bifido and Acidophilus Bacteria in Nutrition and Health," published in the *North European Dairy Journal*, Dr. J.L. Rasic explains, "Changes in the vitamin content occurring during the manufacture of cultured milks are dependent on many factors. Some bacterial strains synthesize vitamins during growth, while others consume them. For instance, yogurt bacteria synthesize folic acid, while acidophilus bacteria consume it. Some yogurts and acidophilus milks are richer in B_{12} and others poorer." The results depend upon the specific strain used when culturing the yogurt. Table 4.3, found on page 46, lists foods in which there is a marked increase in B-complex vitamins as a result of the culturing process.

You should also be aware that all cultured foods are not created equal. For example, simply adding an appropriate amount of acid will result in something that mimics a cultured product. If you have ever added vinegar to plain milk to produce sour milk for a recipe, you understand the process. Some commercial yogurts are made this way. Unfortunately, without the services of the friendly bacteria, products that are directly acidified just aren't as beneficial.

In 1979, the *Journal of Dairy Science* published an article entitled, "Nutritional and Healthful Aspects of Cultured and Cultured-Containing Dairy Products," by Drs. K.M. Shahani and R.C. Chandan. These scientists warn that, "Newer processes have been developed to

Table 4.3 Cultured Foods and B-Complex Vitamin Increase

CULTURED FOOD	B VITAMINS INCREASED
Bifidus milk	B_{12} (cyanocobalamin), Folic acid.
Buttermilk	B_{12} (cyanocobalamin), Folic acid.
Cheddar cheese	B_2 (riboflavin), B_3 (niacin), B_5 (pantothenic acid), B_6 (pyridoxine), Biotin.
Cottage cheese	B_3 (niacin), B_6 (pyridoxine), B_{12} (cyanocobalamin), Biotin, Folic acid.
Kefir	B_{12} (cyanocobalamin), Folic acid.
Sour cream	B_{12} (cyanocobalamin), Folic acid.
Yogurt	B_2 (riboflavin), B_3 (niacin), B_5 (pantothenic acid), B_6 (pyridoxine), B_{12} (cyanocobalamin), Biotin, Folic acid.

manufacture yogurt, cottage cheese, buttermilk, and sour cream by direct acidification instead of by lactic cultures. The advantages of such processes over the conventional culturing methods are (a) elimination of culture-handling problems; (b) better quality control and uniformity of production; and (c) better keeping quality." Drs. Shahani and Chandan emphasize that these commercial benefits are gained at the expense of nutritional value and the loss of the services of the friendly bacteria. For example, instead of folic acid rising to levels of up to 5 micrograms (mcg) per 100 grams in cultured cottage cheese, when processed by direct acidification, the levels rose to only 0.1 mcg—hardly worth measuring.

It's a different story when your friendly bacteria are on the job. The folic acid content of real yogurt, for example, is 3.9 mcg per 100 grams, while the starter milk measures between 0.13 and 0.73 mcg. The friendly bacteria in true yogurt also double the levels of vitamin B_3 (niacin), taking it from between 71 and 96 mcg in the starter milk to between 130 to 141 mcg per 100 grams after culturing. Vitamin A levels in yogurt go up, too. Plain low-fat true yogurt provides between 70 and 130 mcg of vitamin A per 100 grams, but the low-fat starter milk begins with only 9 mcg per 100 grams.

Before culturing, the milk from which cottage cheese is made contains 1 mcg of folic acid per 100 grams. When the culturing process is complete, that level rises to 5 mcg per 100 grams. Cheddar cheese contains up to three times more B_6 than the milk from which it is cultured, with an increase from less than 50 mcg to 147 mcg.

B-complex vitamins are indispensable. They are active in converting carbohydrates into glucose, which your body burns to produce energy. Also needed for the metabolism of fats and proteins, B vitamins are essential for the maintenance of muscle tone in your gastrointestinal tract. They are also necessary for the health of your skin, hair, eyes, mouth, and liver, and they are considered the single most important factor for the healthy maintenance of the nervous system. If you are tired, irritable, nervous, or depressed, or if you suffer from insomnia, neuritis, anemia, or constipation, you may have a vitamin-B deficiency.

THE WEIGHT CONTROL CONNECTION

Those of you who are trying to lose weight probably already know that obesity leads to such conditions as heart disease, kidney trouble, diabetes, high blood pressure, pregnancy difficulties, and even psychological problems. However, you may be surprised to learn that malnutrition is a common cause of obesity. Many overweight people continually eat empty-calorie junk foods instead of the nutrient-rich foods for which their bodies are really hungering. Because they do not supply what the body needs, junk foods are not satisfyingly filling.

Even worse, when you are not taking in the whole nutrients your body requires, fat is not efficiently burned. The production of sufficient energy is the only way to burn fat, and energy production depends on almost every known nutrient, especially high-quality protein and the B-complex vitamins.

Vitamin B_6 (pyridoxine), for instance, is necessary to convert stored fat into an energy source, and it is also a factor in the utilization of proteins. Fat is burned at a greatly reduced rate if the levels of vitamin B_5 (panthothenic acid) and proteins are low. Proteins are needed for the proper functioning of many energy-producing enzymes, and they cannot be broken down without the help of certain other nutrients, including vitamin B_6.

As you have seen, friendly bacteria help with the production of B-complex vitamins and increase the protein content of cultured foods.

Low levels of friendly bacteria make it more difficult to burn off fat and keep it off.

CHOLESTEROL-FIGHTING FRIENDLY BACTERIA

Cholesterol isn't all bad; your body needs some to function properly. It is part and parcel of every cell membrane throughout your body, especially those of the brain, nervous system, liver, and blood. It is needed to form sex and adrenal hormones, vitamin D, and bile, which is necessary for the digestion of fats. Without cholesterol, the normal metabolic processes would be impossible.

Cholesterol is necessary for the metabolism of fats and fat-soluble vitamins. On average, the body manufactures more cholesterol than is contributed by diet, and the manufacturing process is directly tied to the needs of your body. More is produced when your diet is high in fat, especially when those fats are of animal origin.

Bile is manufactured in the liver from some basic raw materials, including cholesterol. Your liver turns the cholesterol into cholic and chenodeoxycholic acids, which are combined with the amino acids glycine and taurine. In this form, bile is stored in your gallbladder and passed into your duodenum after a meal. Bile is an important part of the digestive process of fats. It breaks up fat globules, making them easier to metabolize and digest. Once bile has been used, it is reabsorbed by the small intestine then returned to the liver to be reused.

Before bile can be reabsorbed, it must be broken down again into its basic constituents. Bifidobacteria (and others) have the power to do just that. However, if you are eating a high-fat diet, your liver produces excessive quantities of cholesterol-laden bile. When this happens, many friendly bacteria in your gastrointestinal tract are slowed down or damaged. This is one more good reason for reducing fat in your diet.

A cholesterol problem arises when your levels of low-density lipoproteins (LDLs), better known as the "bad" cholesterol, exceed your needs. On the other hand, high-density lipoproteins (HDLs) actually work to remove excess levels of cholesterol from tissues. This is why, when your cholesterol level is tested, the most important figure is the relationship of HDLs to LDLs, not the total cholesterol count. As long as your HDL levels are high and your LDL levels are low, your risk of suffering a heart attack is minimized.

As you may know, the buildup of plaque in the arteries is one of the main factors involved in atherosclerosis. Heart disease is the number one killer of modern times in Westernized countries. The sticky plaque that builds up on artery walls is made up largely of LDL particles. The higher the levels of LDLs circulating in your bloodstream, the faster atherosclerosis will develop. On the other hand, HDLs are found to be in plentiful supply in people with low levels of "bad" cholesterol, and a low incidence of atherosclerosis. These people are considered to be in good cardiac health.

THE MASAI PHENOMENON

Some people seem to take in large amounts of animal fat without the risk of heart attack. Take the Masai Tribesmen of East Africa. These people—like the Mongols—live a nomadic existence. Their lives depend on the cattle they raise, which they herd from place to place, and their diet is derived entirely from these animals. Like the Mongols, they drink the fermented milk of these animals to which fresh cow blood is added. The cows are regularly bled (not killed) for this purpose.

Although the Masai ingest large amounts of saturated animal fat, their levels of cholesterol are well below those found in most people who eat the average American diet. They also have extremely low levels of heart disease. Although this high-fat diet seems to contradict all that we have been taught, the Masai also have the services of friendly bacteria.

Research shows that the low-risk of heart disease enjoyed by the Masai is due to an anti-cholesterol factor (AMF) found in fermented milk products. This factor has the ability to reduce levels of LDL cholesterol. In spite of many studies, however, the precise "ingredient" responsible has not been identified, but there appear to be two contenders—hydroxymethyglutaric acid and orotic acid. This AMF appears to inhibit the enzyme that synthesizes cholesterol. Similar anticholesterol effects have been demonstrated in live yogurt.

Fermentation does not seem to be the essential factor in producing the AMF effect. Studies show it is present in sweet acidophilus milk, which is not fermented. The degree of concentration required to produce the AMF effect, according to Dr. Khem Shahani, is 4 million viable acidophilus organisms per milliliter of milk. The *Lactobacillus acidophilus* super strain that produces this anticholesterol effect is DDS-1.

SCIENCE SAYS

Studies in both animals and humans have shown that cultured milk products to which acidophilus cultures have been added—including yogurt and sweet acidophilus milk—efficiently lower levels of cholesterol in the blood. In a number of studies in which rats, pigs, and rabbits were fed *L. acidophilus*, these animals showed a dramatic reduction in blood cholesterol levels.

These studies showed that the ability to reduce cholesterol levels is directly tied to specific super strains of acidophilus. For example, one acidophilus super strain, RP32, broke down cholesterol easily in an oxygen-free environment, such as that found in the large intestine. Another study using an acidophilus strain designated as P47 failed to do so. The strain is an all-important factor.

The friendly bacteria found in certain super strains have the ability to break down bile. When animals are kept "germ-free," with no colonization of beneficial bacteria or other flora in their gastrointestinal tracts, it has been shown that their bile remains unchanged from that which the animal produces for the digestion of fats. It cannot be recycled in this form. When suitable bacterial cultures, such as bifidobacteria and acidophilus, were given to these same "germ-free" animals, their bile was either recycled back to the liver or exited the body in changed form. The action of the beneficial bacteria on bile somehow removed the cholesterol from the systems of these animals.

It seems as if the friendly bacteria simply "ate" the cholesterol. Dr. S.E. Gilliland and his colleagues reported on their study in a paper entitled, "Assimilation of Cholesterol by *Lactobacillus Acidophilus*," published in the February 1985 issue of *Applied and Environmental Microbiology*.

Dr. Gilliland showed that when acidophilus was grown in the presence of cholesterol, some cholesterol actually appeared inside the lactobacillus cells while they were growing. The scientists were able to confirm this effect by a reduction in the amount of cholesterol present in the surrounding growth medium. Dr. Gilliland stressed that the amount of cholesterol added to the culture dishes was not in excess of quantities normally found in the intestines. This effect occurred only when bile was present but there was no oxygen—the precise conditions found in the gastrointestinal tract.

The conclusion reached by Dr. Gilliland was that this ability of *Lactobacillus acidophilus*, "would make it possible for the organism to assimilate at least part of the cholesterol ingested in the diet, making it unavailable for absorption into the blood." A similar action could be expected on cholesterol that is manufactured in the human body.

This effect was confirmed in 1979, when the *American Journal of Clinical Nutrition* published a paper by G. Hepner entitled "Hypocholesterolemic Effect of Yogurt and Milk." Dr. Hepner reported on a study involving fifty-four volunteers between the ages of twenty-one and fifty-five who were studied for twelve weeks. All of the subjects were in good health and had no history of cardiovascular or gallbladder disease. During the first four and last four weeks of the study, they were given either unpasteurized yogurt, pasteurized yogurt, or milk. Both forms of the yogurt contained cultures of *Lactobacillus bulgaricus* and *Streptococcus thermophilus.*

The volunteers were asked not to make any changes in their diets or lifestyle choices (twelve were smokers) or alter their routines in any way. During the length of the study, a great deal of detailed information was taken from each subject. Individual nutritional patterns were recorded and blood constituents were monitored constantly. There was no significant alteration in the total calorie intake, or in the amount of cholesterol, protein, carbohydrates, fat, or fiber that each subject consumed. Dr. Hepner wanted to make sure that any changes in the blood cholesterol levels of each person came about as a result of the yogurt supplementation, rather than any dietary restrictions.

What he found confirmed all the laboratory studies. Decreased cholesterol levels in the blood were apparent within seven days of yogurt intake. Each person who ingested live yogurt benefited, some more than others. Dr. Hepner recorded a reduction of between 5 and 10 percent in cholesterol levels in each volunteer on the live yogurt regimen. These beneficial results continued for four weeks after the yogurt was withdrawn, showing that the transient yogurt bacteria remained in the gastrointestinal tract for that period of time.

Dr. Hepner and his colleagues referred to similar studies in their paper. For example, one such study showed that when yogurt was supplemented in very large amounts of up to nearly half the daily calorie intake, there was a substantial reduction in cholesterol levels among healthy volunteers. This study also showed that the synthesis of cholesterol in the body was slowed down during the course of yogurt supplementation.

YOUR FRIENDLY BACTERIA AT WORK

The researchers came to no firm conclusions in any of the studies cited above. However, they did theorize that the decrease in blood cholesterol levels in subjects given live yogurt could be the result of an alteration in cholesterol synthesis, increased absorption, conversion of cholesterol into bile acids, or the initial synthesis and breakdown of lipoproteins.

In 1975, Dr. M.L. Speck's paper, "Interactions Among Lactobacilli and Man," was published by the *Journal of Dairy Science*. Dr. Speck showed that when bile is broken down into its constituents, the resulting free acids have an inhibitory effect on the growth and activity of rival organisms. As a result of the breakdown of bile salts, which in itself leads to a lowering of cholesterol levels, the normal passage of certain of these acids in the circulation between the liver and the gastrointestinal tract continues.

In his paper, "Lactobacilli and Human Health," Dr. C.S. Hangee-Bauer of Bastyr College states, "There are a variety of mechanisms to explain the apparent hypocholesterolemic [anti-cholesterol] results of lactobacillus fermentation. Lactobacilli may metabolize cholesterol for energy, suggesting that cholesterol may be a 'food' for this organism. Other possibilities include an alteration in the bile acid metabolism due to modification of the bowel flora, which would favor increased excretion of cholesterol (and other factors)."

To put it more simply, various studies show two ways your friendly bacteria help reduce cholesterol in the blood. The first is by breaking it down for easy removal, and the second is by directly absorbing it.

CONCLUSION

I have explained how your friendly bacteria increase the protein value of high-quality foods that are protein-rich even before they come in contact with the friendly bacteria. You have seen how beneficial bacteria aid in the digestion of milk products, increase the bioavailability of both calcium and protein, and alter cholesterol. However, you should also remember that the cholesterol-fighting effects of the friendly bacteria do not give you complete protection against the documented risks that come from eating a high-fat diet. You still must do your part, which includes enlisting the aid of friendly bacteria.

Health truly does begin within, but unless you make sure your gastrointestinal tract really does have beneficial bacteria, everything you learn in this book will be a waste of information. A bowl of live yogurt in your refrigerator or a probiotic supplement on your breakfast table won't do you a bit of good until you consume one or the other, or, preferably, both.

Now that you've seen how the friendly bacteria help with your nutrient needs, in the next chapter, you'll see how the youngest members of the family can benefit. Newborns and children need friendly bacteria, too, perhaps most of all.

5

Babies and Friendly Bacteria

Most babies born to healthy mothers come into the world clean. However, within a few days of birth, your baby's gastrointestinal tract will be colonized by bacteria. How your child was born—vaginally or by cesarean section—strongly influences the type of bacteria your infant will carry. For example, early studies show that *Bifidobacteria infantis* was once found in approximately 60 percent of four- to six-day old full-term babies who were born vaginally. In contrast, only 9 percent of babies born by cesarean section were colonized with *B. infantis*. Through a mysterious phenomenon of Mother Nature, babies pick up friendly bacteria from their mothers during their passage through a clean and healthy birth canal.

We have known for centuries that a healthy mother is more likely to bring forth a healthy baby. In addition to eating right, exercising, taking vitamins, refraining from smoking or drinking, and receiving adequate prenatal care, pregnant women, as well as nursing mothers and infants, also need probiotic supplements. In this chapter, you will learn why.

UNBORN BABIES AND BACTERIA

Current research shows that a bacterial or yeast infection in the vaginal tract can have extremely serious affects on an unborn child, including triggering a premature birth. In her 1994 paper, "Microbiology of Obstetric and Gynecologic Infections," Dr. Hannah Wexler says,

"Infections of the female genital tract cause considerable morbidity; costs, both economic and human, are staggering. Bacterial vaginitis and vaginosis alone are responsible for approximately 10 million office visits per year and may be associated with a variety of more serious conditions, including postpartum endometrititis, pelvic cellulitis, pelvic inflammatory disease, and chorioamnionitis." Chorioamnionitis is an inflammation of the amniotic sac that protects the fetus. It is caused by organisms in the fluid surrounding the fetus within the amniotic sac.

To understand the cause of many obstetric and gynecologic infections, you should first know that friendly lactobacteria maintain control of the normal vaginal ecology. In so doing, they provide an important defense against colonization by dangerous organisms. Dr. Wexler explains, "Bacterial vaginosis has been described as a microecologic shift in the dominant organism of the microecology from *L. acidophilus* to *Gardnerella vaginalis*, resulting in favorable conditions for the establishment of anaerobic flora. Production of hydrogen peroxide (H_2O_2) and bacteriocins, and a lower pH are all thought to play a role in the protective nature of this organism [*L. acidophilus*]. The role of H_2O_2 is thought to be critical in controlling genital microflora; in a study of pregnant women, those colonized by H_2O_2-positive lactobacilli were less likely to have bacterial vaginosis, symptomatic candidiasis, and vaginal colonization by *G. vaginalis, Bacteroides sp., Peptostreptococcus sp., Mycoplasma hominis, Ureaplasma urealyticum,* and *Veridians streptococci.* Women without vaginal lactobacilli were more likely than women with H_2O_2-producing lactobacilli to have these same organisms, as well as *Chlamydia trachomatis.*"

Dr. Wexler warns, "Although bacterial vaginosis is not a direct health threat [to the mother], the opportunistic pathogens present in this condition place the woman at higher risk for other more serious infections. Bacterial vaginosis has been linked to a wide variety of upper genital tract infections, including clinical chorioamnionitis, preterm delivery, and postpartum and post-surgical infections (postpartum endometritis, post-hysterectomy vaginal cuff cellulitis, and postabortion pelvic inflammatory disease)."

In one part of this study, Dr. Wexler selected 171 pregnant women to examine. At term, each woman's vaginal flora was rated on the basis of a vaginal smear. The flora was considered normal when lactobacteria predominated in the vaginal tract (50 percent), intermediate when there was a fair amount of lactobacteria present (27 percent), or contaminated when the vaginal tract had only a small amount of lactobacteria (23 percent) and bacterial vaginosis was diagnosed. Dr. Wexler determined that high concentrations of opportunistic pathogenic bacteria in the lower genital tract place women—especially pregnant women—at increased risk for genital infections and adverse pregnancy outcomes.

She writes, "Considerable information links vaginosis with preterm premature rupture of the membranes, as well as with pre-term labor and birth. High concentrations of vaginal microorganisms have been associated with an increased rate of pre-term delivery. . . . High levels of facultative lactobacilli . . . were associated with a decreased rate of pre-term delivery. . . ."

If you are beginning to think that your baby might fare better if he or she is delivered by cesarean section, that is not necessarily so. Dr. Wexler states, "Postcesarean section endometritis and postoperative cuff cellulitis both involve the ascent of potentially pathogenic organisms found in the vagina, and vaginosis appears to be a risk factor for the development of these infections. The bacteria may contaminate the endometrial cavity during delivery; during cesarean section, these bacteria gain access to the uterine incision, the pelvic peritoneum, and the abdominal wound."

It has been only in the last several years that medical science has pieced together the relationship between the presence of the friendly bacteria in the birth canal and healthy, full-term babies. The facts are clear. Fortunately, pregnant women can avoid all these complications by taking supplemental probiotics daily. By protecting their own health, mothers-to-be also protect that of their unborn children.

One Swedish study entitled, "Bacterial Vaginosis and Vaginal Microorganisms in Idiopathic Premature Labor and Association with Pregnancy Outcome," published in the January 1994 issue of the *Journal of Clinical Microbiology*, showed that a vaginal infection is often a causative factor in premature and low birth weight infants. This study of the vaginal microflora of 49 women in preterm labor was compared with the flora of 38 term controls to discover if the presence of specific microorganisms in the vagina influenced the rate of premature births. What this work confirmed is that vaginal infections in pregnant women present a risk to the fetus. The researchers point out that only 7 percent of all deliveries are preterm, but these premature births account for more than 80 percent of deaths occurring in babies in the first month of life. The study concludes with this statement, "Our study clearly indicates that BV [bacterial vaginosis] and its associated organisms are correlated with idiopathic premature delivery." For information on how friendly bacteria can help relieve vaginal infections, see Vaginitis in Part Two.

BABY BACTERIA

As its name implies, *Bifidobacteria infantis* is a natural inhabitant of the gastrointestinal tract of human infants. It also occurs in small numbers in the female vagina, along with *L. acidophilus*. The bifidobacteria, including *B. infantis, B. bifidum, B. longum, and B. breve*, are the predominant bacteria in the large intestines of babies. They are special varieties, not the same strains found in adults. These bacteria are considered "anaerobic;" they do not require oxygen. They produce acetic and lactic acids, plus small amounts of formic acid, from carbohydrates. The major beneficial functions of the "baby bacteria" are similar to those of bifidobacteria in adults discussed in Chapter 3.

The common strains of baby bifidobacteria prevent the colonization of invading pathogens in your infant's intestine because they are fierce competitors for nutrients and attachment sites along the intestinal wall. When sufficient numbers of baby bifidobacteria are in residence, the bad bacteria can't find room to colonize. The production of acetic and lactic acids by the bifidobacteria increases the acidity of the intestine, further inhibiting the growth of undesirable bacteria. These friendly bacteria also assist in nitrogen retention, assuring normal weight gain in infants. Like their "big brothers," baby bifidos inhibit the bacteria that converts nitrates into the potentially harmful carcinogenic nitrites. And, of course, they produce those very important B-complex vitamins.

THE BACTERIA IN BREAST MILK

Once upon a time, breast milk was considered the best food for infants. In some circles, it is still so regarded. However, even Nature's perfect food source has become tainted by the damage we have done to the ecology of our planet.

There is evidence that the quality of breast milk has declined worldwide, almost certainly because of the manmade pollutants found in the air, water, and food chain. The intestinal flora of babies today is far different from that of infants less than half a century ago. Although *B. infantis* is the preferred colonizer, more recent investigations show that other species of bifidobacteria, such as *B. bifidum* and *B. longum*, are now dominant in the colonies of breastfed babies.

Does it matter? Oh, yes, very much so. In 1988, in a paper entitled, "Occurrence of *B. infantis* and *B. bifidum* in the Gut of Infants and Adults," Dr. J.L. Rasic reported on a German study that focused on the composition of intestinal flora in infants for nearly thirty years. This study showed a measurable decline in both the numbers of and changes in the strains of bifidobacteria found in breastfed babies. The *decline* in beneficial bacteria was accompanied by a *rise* in the levels of undesirable pathogenic organisms. Between 1974 and 1977—the final years of the study—the researchers found that more than 10 percent of the babies examined had no bifidobacteria in their stool.

A similar trend was observed in premature babies studied over the same time frame. Although premature infants have a naturally lower concentration of bifidobacteria than full-term babies, even lower levels of bifidobacteria were documented in this more fragile group of newborns.

Dr. Rasic reports that he has found steadily increasing levels of *Klebsiella* and certain pathogenic strains of *E. coli*, both potentially very dangerous bacteria, in these same babies. These species of disease-causing bacteria are now commonly found to be resistant to antibiotics. Dr. Rasic has also observed a gradual rise in the average levels of pH in the gastrointestinal tract of babies, indicating lower levels of acidity in the large intestine. This factor is known to promote the overgrowth of undesirable bacteria and fungi.

Researchers in Britain, Germany, and France have confirmed Dr. Rasic's findings. Using computer models, a group of scientists has predicted that babies are faced with a steady loss of beneficial bacteria, accompanied, inevitably, by an increase in the levels of dangerous disease-causing microorganisms in their bowels. The consequences of this shift in bacterial populations could be very serious.

Drs. A. Schecter and T. Gasiewicz outlined the problem in their 1987 book, *Solving Hazardous Waste Problems*. They documented the high levels of toxic chemicals such as polychlorinated dibenzo-p-doxin (PCDD) and polychlorinated dibenzofurans (PCDF) in human breast milk in such diverse geographical locations as the United States, Canada, and Vietnam. Breastfed infants are on the front line for receiving these toxins. Understandably, levels of toxic breast milk were much higher in Vietnam because of the herbicides dropped during the Vietnam War. However, levels of these potentially cancer-causing chemicals also have been found in the breast milk of North American mothers.

A consequence of the spraying that took place in Vietnam, dioxins and furans are also found in such sources as common garden pesticides, wood preservatives, certain household paper products, and the emissions from incinerators. These dangerous chemicals have been discovered in atmospheric pollution, tainted water, and seafood that comes from contaminated oceans, rivers, and lakes.

Dr. Schecter and his colleagues recommend the long-term observation of babies fed contaminated breast milk. They cite that these chemicals are especially worrisome because they have been known to cause cancer in animal studies.

In a *USA Today* article published in December 1987, Dr. Philip Anderson of the University of California, an authority on tainted breast milk, is quoted as saying, "The longer they breast-feed, the more [toxins] the babies get. We cannot permit the contamination of our most precious resource to continue." That was almost ten years ago. The problem is worse today.

Be that as it may, I must emphasize that I am not suggesting that a new mother opt for formula over breast milk, if she is able to nurse her child. The very first milk a nursing mother gives her baby is colostrum. Colostrum contains water, protein, fats, and carbohydrates, plus important substances that fight hostile bacteria, including white blood cells that provide a boost to the infant's young immune system. These substances encourage the development of bifidobacteria colonies, which, in turn, increase the acidity of the colonized region and create a hostile environment for harmful bacteria.

In any case, formula-fed infants face another set of problems. In both instances, the problem is a deficiency of beneficial bacteria.

FORMULA-FED INFANTS

The most obvious difference between breastfed and formula-fed infants is the makeup of the child's stool. Babies on breast milk have loose stools with a rather "cheesy" odor, and an acid pH. Most formula-fed babies produce feces that are almost adult in odor, appearance, and composition, if not in size. The pH level is the same, too, between 6.0 and 7.0.

In 1980, the *American Journal of Clinical Nutrition* published a paper entitled, "Influence of Breast Feeding on Bifido Flora of the Newborn Intestine," by Drs. H. Beerens, C. Romond, and C. Neut. These doctors reported that the numbers of bifidobacteria in groups of differently fed infants may appear similar, but the species differ. They warn that this difference carries with it serious health implications.

This study showed that the main difference between infants fed cow's milk and those fed breast milk is the presence of high levels of dangerous *Bacteroides*, *Clostridium*, and *E. coli* in the babies fed cow's milk. These levels do not decrease as the child gets older.

After examining a variety of possible food sources that might enhance the colonization of the infant's gastrointestinal tract with beneficial bacteria, the doctors concluded that human breast milk is still best. They state, "None of the other mammalian milks favored the growth of bifidobacteria species (*B. infantis*, *B. bifidum*, and *B. longum*). This suggests the presence [in human breast milk] of a specific factor that we have termed the 'BB factor.'" Although the doctors did not identify the substance in human milk that stimulates bifidobacteria growth; they did state that the substance is heat-stable and not a protein.

Manufacturers of infant formulas try very hard to provide the constituents of human breast milk in their product, but they fail. Formulas based largely on cow's milk, as well as soy formulas, simply cannot sustain those vitally important bifidobacteria colonies in a baby's bowel.

BIFIDOBACTERIA AND YOUR BABY

Dr. J.L. Rasic points to a growing decline in beneficial bacteria, such as *B. infantis*, that can prevent infant diarrhea, and an increase in the harmful bacteria that cause it. Uncontrollable diarrhea is one of the major causes of infant death. This is likely to happen especially when a baby has suffered through several episodes of ill health or is malnourished to begin with. Although diarrhea is still most prevalent in Third World and underdeveloped countries, it remains a major cause of death in industrialized countries as well. Over 1,000 children under the age of twelve months die each year in the United States from the effects of diarrhea.

The harmful bacteria most often involved in this sort of intestinal illness are certain strains of *E. coli*, which attack either the small or large intestine, where they do their damage by producing toxins. The intestines can also be invaded by various strains of *Salmonella*. This bacteria attaches itself to the mucous membranes and penetrates them. Once this is achieved, it creates havoc by directly spreading into other areas. In the large intestine, *Shigella* produces symptoms through direct invasion and/or toxin production.

These and other pathogens are controlled by healthy flora when your child's gastrointestinal tract is well colonized by bifidobacteria strains, such as *B. infantis*. Unfortunately, this particular bacteria is on the decline. As we have seen, a decline in *B. infantis* is always accompanied by a rise in dangerous bacteria.

Dr. J.L. Rasic explains that *B. infantis* is less "robust" than the other bifidobacteria, meaning that it is less able to cope with the growing worldwide contaminants found in the food chain, air, and water. Nonetheless, *B. infantis* is able to cope with those dangerous invading microorganisms, including *E. coli*, *Klebsiella*, and even *Salmonella*.

Friendly bacteria bring the same benefits to babies that they bring to you. Calcium absorption is enhanced by the presence of the friendly, acid-producing bacteria. Friendly bacteria also aid in the digestion of milk sugars and increase the digestibility of proteins. Dr. Rasic has found that when underweight infants are given supplements of *B. infantis*, there is an increase in nitrogen retention, which helps the child achieve normal weight gain. Bifidobacteria deliver B-complex vitamins, as well. These are all very important benefits for newborns.

PROBIOTICS FOR INFANTS

By now, you are well-acquainted with both the bifido and lacto families of friendly bacteria. Perhaps you are wondering why *L. bulgaricus* and *L. acidophilus* have not been discussed in this chapter. I have told you that the friendly bacteria do the same things for babies as they do for adults. However, here again, the species and strain are all-important. Some strains of these microorganisms produce the D form of lactic acid instead of the L form. While either strain is beneficial for adults, the D form of lactic acid is poorly tolerated by infants' digestive tracts.

Streptococcus faecium is another common inhabitant of the gastrointestinal tract that, in some cases, assists bifidobacteria by contributing large quantities of acetic acid to the area. However, some strains of this particular bacteria have the ability to cause food poisoning. Most are safe, according to research, but some are not. You should be aware that some manufacturers include large amounts of *E. faecium*, formerly known as *S. faecium*, in their supplemental lactobacillus mixtures, mainly because these cultures are significantly cheaper and easier to grow than the better known lactobacteria.

In a paper entitled, "Factors Affecting Enterotoxin Production by Thermonuclease Positive *Streptococcus faecium* SF-100 Isolated from an Infant Food," published in *The Journal of Food Science* in 1985, Drs. V.K. Batish, H. Chander, and B. Ranjanathan showed that in a slightly alkaline environment at a temperature of 98.6°F (37 °C), dangerous enterotoxins produced by the SF-100 strain of *S. faecium* were at their maximum production after eight hours. Should this strain find its way into an infant's digestive tract that is not well-colonized with friendly bacteria, there is the real possibility of harm.

E. faecium has also become resistant to vancomycin, one of the last remaining "big guns" of the antibiotic family. Even worse, this bacteria has the ability to transfer this characteristic to other dangerous bacteria. This means that the body of anyone ingesting *E. faecium* could become a production facility for drug-resistant bacteria. When this news broke, at least two manufacturers stopped using *E. faecium* in their supplemental lactobacillus mixtures.

My advice is to give your child *B. infantis* only. Unless you have consulted with a knowledgeable health care professional who knows the importance of strains regarding the use of *L. bulgaricus*, *L. acidophilus* and/or *E. faecium* for your baby, you should steer clear of these supplements.

CONCLUSION

There is no need to deny your baby the proven benefits of probiotic supplementation; however, we live in an increasingly polluted world. Baby bacteria are declining, while dangerous drug-resistant bacteria are increasing. All babies—whether breast-fed or bottle-fed—need the protection of friendly bacteria. Remember that *B. infantis* is Nature's choice for babies, and should be yours as well. This "infant bacteria" is safe for babies. The Malyoth strain of *B. bifidum* can assist in the repopulation of your baby's gastrointestinal tract with friendly bacteria, too.

And, if you are a pregnant mother-to-be, here's a special reminder. Whether your child is born vaginally or by cesarean section, he or she will arrive clean, healthy, and free of bacterial contamination as long as you are. The health of your unborn child begins within *you*.

6

The Foes of
Friendly Bacteria

*T*here are a number of factors, both internal and external, that make a dramatic impact on the overall level of health and well being of your beneficial bacteria. You should know that both over-the-counter and prescription drugs, including antibiotics, cortisone, and birth control pills, wear down the normal levels of beneficial bacteria in your intestines. Radiation and chemotherapy treatments, environmental pollutants, food additives, alcohol, tobacco smoke, stress, and strong herbs also impact friendly bacteria negatively. What you eat or don't eat is another critical factor. And measurable amounts of beneficial bacteria are lost as a natural part of the aging process.

Under ideal conditions, such as in a petri dish with no competing microorganisms, bacteria—both good and bad—have the ability to divide every twenty minutes to form two new microorganisms. This means that by the end of an eight-hour period, one lonesome bacteria can produce about 42.5 million microorganisms all by itself.

Fortunately, there are two factors working in our favor. First, the friendly bacteria are fierce competitors. They work hard to keep the environment decidedly unfriendly to interlopers. When the gastrointestinal tract is adequately colonized with the good guys, harmful bacteria don't stand much of a chance.

Second—and this applies to both good and bad bacteria—ideal conditions for replication do not exist inside any one of us. If our bodies were ideal breeding grounds, the human body would be overwhelmed by the sheer volume of these organisms. Experts say that it is more likely that each bacteria in the gastrointestinal tract divides no more than four times and likely only once every twenty-four hours. If we're discussing harmful bacteria, that's good, of course. However, if we're talking about friendly bacteria, that's bad.

This chapter addresses the factors that can negatively impact your beneficial bacteria. For the most part, these factors include the use of antacids, antibiotics, laxatives, and estrogen; poor dietary choices; and the engagement in anal intercourse. These factors are largely under your personal control.

USE OF ANTACIDS

The acidic secretions produced in your stomach are necessary to the digestive process. In addition, proper acid levels keep the harmful bacterial population of the stomach and small intestine under control. Whenever acid production slows down, for whatever reason, the shift to alkaline pH levels fosters the buildup of undesirable bacteria and an overgrowth of *Candida albicans*—a tenacious yeast that changes into a fungus that can cause serious consequences to your health.

Antacids are designed to neutralize and/or absorb the acid secretions of the digestive tract, but hydrochloric acid is a major player in your gastric juices. Necessary for the proper digestion of food, hydrochloric acid also destroys harmful bacteria that would otherwise escape into your intestines. The frequent use of antacids—including that old standby, bicarbonate of soda—quickly shifts the acid environment to an alkaline one, which is highly favorable for harmful bacteria.

There are other negative effects linked to the overuse of antacids. Those that contain magnesium tend to have a laxative effect. And many antacids contain aluminum salts (including aluminum hydroxychloride), which are drying agents found in many antiperspirants, antiseptics, astringents, and styptics. Although the evidence isn't conclusive, aluminum has been implicated in the development of Alzheimer's disease. Also, antacids formulated with aluminum and calcium are known to cause constipation.

USE OF LAXATIVES

Bowel movements depend on peristaltic action to move things

along. This rhythmical contraction of the muscles lining the walls of the small intestine helps prevent undesirable bacterial colonies from setting up residence there. Peristaltic action, coupled with thriving colonies of friendly bacteria, make your small intestine a decidedly inhospitable place for dangerous bacteria that are seeking a niche to colonize. When peristaltic action slows down, a rapid overgrowth of harmful bacteria is not only possible, but probable. The situation turns serious when the friendly bacteria aren't up to strength; dangerous organisms take advantage of the situation and move right in.

The overuse of laxatives is the most common reason for reduced peristaltic action. When the body becomes dependent on the artificial stimulation that laxatives provide, the intestines become lazy and "forget" their responsibility. Unless a diseased state exists to explain slow (or nonexistent) peristalsis, a diet rich in fruits, whole grains, vegetables, and lots of pure water is the best way to correct the problem. It is not a coincidence that these same dietary recommendations are the heart of a bifidogenic diet, which supports the care and feeding of your friendly bacteria.

Those who experience constipation due to laxative overuse should strengthen their friendly bacteria by taking supplementary probiotics. This is the best way to make sure harmful bacteria that find their way into your intestines are not able to find an attachment site and are forced to move on.

HOSTILE BACTERIAL INTERACTION

The interaction of one type of bacteria with another is very important in determining the pattern of colonization that develops in your gastrointestinal tract. Unless oxygen-dependent bacteria are present in sufficient numbers to reduce oxygen levels in an area, the bacteria that require an oxygen-free environment, such as bifidobacteria, cannot survive in abundant good health.

Secretions of various bacteria—both friendly and unfriendly—also play a part in determining who survives and who doesn't. The friendly bacteria are noted acid producers, which is one way they keep harmful bacteria and opportunistic organisms (like yeast) that require a more alkaline environment from proliferating.

POOR DIETARY CHOICES

Food choices can make a difference in the balance of power in the nev-erending bacterial wars that are waged in your intestinal tract. In short-term studies, the change is measurable. In long-term studies, it is dramatic.

The very young undergo relatively swift changes in their resident intestinal bacteria. For example, the intestines of a breastfed infant are generally populated with a large number of beneficial bifidobacteria. However, during the period when a child is being weaned from the breast, a gradual increase in the number of putrefactive bacteria occurs until the balance of power becomes even. Mixtures of bacteri-al flora appear in the child's colon, including *clostridium*, *E. coli*, and *streptococcus*.

Dietary changes that alter the metabolic activity of bifidobacteria, even though they may remain at the same population level, reduce the ability of the friendly bacteria to produce the volatile fatty acids they need to control harmful bacteria. This allows harmful bacteria to become more active and do more damage, even though the good guys are still high in numbers.

In the short term, even though the levels of the different inhabitants of the gastrointestinal tract don't shift much according to what you eat, the way in which they react within their closed environment changes greatly. In other words, although dietary choices may not immediately change the balance of power in your gastrointestinal tract, your diet very definitely changes the way these bacteria interact with each other by altering the types of substances they secrete.

Over the long term, it's a very different story. Drs. G.L. Simon and S.L. Gorbach, who contributed a chapter entitled, "Intestinal Flora in Health and Disease," to the book *Physiology of the Gastrointestinal Tract*, write, "Studies of metabolic activity of the flora based on measure-ments of bacterial enzymes have in fact revealed marked changes in the colonic flora as a function of diet."

As discussed earlier, dietary choices impact your overall health and well being. A diet high in fat and red meat leads to high levels of harmful bacteria, as well as potentially carcinogenic substances that linger in your intestines. On the other hand, a high-carbohydrate, bifi-dogenic diet reduces the metabolic mischief perpetrated by danger-ous microorganisms. In one study, simply adding sweet acidophilus milk to the diet of research subjects led to an increase in the numbers of the friendly bacteria, which, in turn, led to a measurable reduction of the undesirables in the neighborhood. If a glass of acidophilus or bifidus milk or a bowl of real yogurt can do all that—and they can— think of how much more probiotic supplements containing billions of viable friendly bacteria can do for you.

ANAL INTERCOURSE

Anal intercourse—heterosexual or homosexual—can cause overwhelming damage to the lower bowel. This sensitive region is traumatized by this form of sexual behavior, resulting in lacerations and abrasions that make it easy for infectious bacteria to create havoc.

Anal intercourse is known to foster multiple infections by introducing a host of bacteria, viruses, protozoa, parasites, and yeast into a region that is not equipped to deal with such invasions. Most often, these invaders overwhelm the friendly bacteria, resulting in chronic hard-to-treat infections.

Certain factors common in anal intercourse cause a lowering of immune function. For instance, the anal area, unlike the vaginal region, is not self-lubricating, so petroleum jelly is often used to facilitate anal intercourse. Petrochemical-based lubricants are strongly immunosuppressive. Also, introducing sperm into the colon is risky as sperm itself suppresses the immune function. If sperm didn't have the ability to "turn off" the immune system and bypass the protective bacteria residing in the female vagina, they would be destroyed before they could reach their objective.

In short, anal intercourse severely disturbs the bowel's ecology, resulting in a marked lowering of immune function, both locally and generally. Those who indulge in this practice face a wide range of problems, including serious infections and nutritional deficiencies that come about when the intestines cannot perform normally. Yes, the assistance friendly bacteria can provide is considerable, but it's not enough to repair localized damage.

USE OF ANTIBIOTICS

Almost any antibiotic will alter the bacterial balance in your intestines. If you've ever had an operation, you probably know that antibiotics are often administered before surgery, especially abdominal surgery, to minimize the likelihood of a post-operative infection.

Data collected from veterans' hospitals throughout the United States show that the use of antibiotics before surgery results in both aerobic and anaerobic bacterial levels dropping to between 20 and 25 percent of their original levels. This leads to a documented reduction in post-operative infections. Only 9 percent of those who received pre-operative antibiotics developed bacterial infections, compared to 35 percent of those who were not given antibiotics.

That's the good news. However, as I have frequently told you, antibiotics cause a massive die-off of most of the bacteria in the body, including the beneficial friendly bacteria. Because more and more drug-resistant bacteria have appeared on the scene, the so-called "big guns" of the antibiotic arsenal are the ones most frequently prescribed today. These broad-spectrum antibiotics hit friend and foe indiscriminately. The ecological vacuum created by the destruction of your friendly bacteria is often rapidly filled by potentially pathogenic microorganisms. With billions of attachment sites open, dangerous bacteria have the opportunity to move right in.

The rapid repopulation of the gastrointestinal tract by "bad guys" after antibiotic therapy are numerous and common. For example, the overgrowth of the particularly dangerous organism *Clostridium dificile* gives rise to a condition called *Pseudomembranous enterocolitis*. The end result of the toxins produced by this opportunistic invader is serious. With symptoms that include bloody diarrhea, pain, and catastrophic weight loss, this bacteria causes ulcers that destroy the intestinal lining.

Another pathogenic bacteria that is known to take advantage of residential openings created by the loss of friendly bacteria after the use of broad-spectrum antibiotics is *Staphlyococcus aureus*. Overgrowth of this bacteria produces symptoms that are similar to enterocolitis produced by *Clostridium dificile.*

Super-infections are another possible result of antibiotic treatment. Remember, while many friendly and unfriendly bacteria are destroyed, there are a number of drug-resistant pathogens that live on. These surviving powerful drug-resistant bacteria have an unobstructed playing field. The microorganisms most frequently implicated in super-infections include *staphylococcus, pseudomonas,* and certain proteus species. And super-infections that follow antibiotic therapy are not limited to your gastrointestinal tract; they can occur in almost any region or organ of your body.

When your friendly bacterial forces have been decimated by antibiotics, other unfriendly bacteria, yeast, and fungi already living in your intestines (and once under the tight control of the friendly bacteria) are free to proliferate wildly. The overgrowth of one particularly strong parasitic yeastlike fungus—*Candida albicans*—results in a serious condition called candidiasis. Depending on its location, symptoms of candidiasis may include inflammation of the tongue, mouth, or rectum; vaginitis; and a range of mental and emotional symptoms such as anxiety, irritability, and even depression. Multiple allergies that manifest themselves as digestive disorders, such as bloating, heartburn, constipation, and diarrhea, also have been tied to yeast overgrowth. Cystitis, premenstrual syndrome, fatigue, and acne and other skin problems are also implicated in a candida outbreak of long duration. Because of its many and varied symptoms, candidiasis is often misdiagnosed. (For more information, see Candidiasis in Part Two.)

I am not saying you should never take antibiotics. There may very well come a time when they are necessary. Just remember that you are more in need of probiotics when you are taking antibiotics than at any other time. Taking daily supplemental friendly bacteria is the best way to insure the strength of your first line of defense.

REDUCED ESTROGEN LEVELS

Sex hormones have an important relationship with the bacteria in your gastrointestinal tract. When a healthy female body is functioning normally, over 60 percent of the female hormones, including estrogen, are passed into the intestines in bile fluids. Although a small amount of estrogen is excreted in fecal matter, the majority of the female sex hormones are processed by bacterial enzymes before they are reabsorbed into the bloodstream. In a healthy body, the hormones are routed through the blood back to the liver for reactivation into a biologically active form the body can use.

Some estrogen is chemically changed by the mucosal cells of the bowel into a form that cannot be recycled via the liver. This form is excreted in the urine. Since the process leading to urinary excretion can take place only in the lining of the colon, the levels of estrogen found in urine can determine the efficiency of the processes that take place in the gastrointestinal tract. Antibiotics and oral contraceptives chemically change the way in which the female body deals with estrogen.

When antibiotics are taken, the levels of estrogen found in the urine are much lower than normal. In addition, the levels of reabsorbed and recycled estrogen are also much lower. For example, the quantities of this important female hormone found in fresh feces rises to as much as sixty times the normal levels during antibiotic therapy. These changes in hormone levels are believed to be the result from the damage done to the friendly bacteria by antibiotic use.

There are numerous documented cases of women who have gotten pregnant while taking both oral contraceptives and antibiotics. This is because the circulating levels of sex hormones are reduced due to the effect of antibiotics on the friendly bacteria. Most women who take birth control pills while taking prescribed antibiotics are advised by their doctors to abstain from sexual intercourse during treatment, and to allow sufficient time to pass after the treatment is completed for their hormone levels to return to normal.

Reduced estrogen levels are implicated in a number of other conditions, including breakthrough bleeding during the quiet time of the menstrual cycle, and the development of osteoporosis.

The best way to prevent antibiotics from disturbing estrogen levels is by taking probiotic supplements daily. This will keep the gastrointestinal tract densely colonized with much-needed friendly bacteria.

CONCLUSION

By and large, you have the ability to avoid these foes of your friendly bacteria. This is an important responsibility in maintaining strong armies of friendly bacteria—your first line of defense against illness.

7

The Antibiotic Action
of Friendly Bacteria

The term *antibiotic* refers to the ability of a substance to kill or prevent the growth of a living organism. Because bacteria and microbes are living organisms, substances primarily known as antibiotics also encompass antibacterial and antimicrobial substances. Basically, whether a drug or substance is labeled antibiotic, antibacterial, or antimicrobial, all three substances do the same thing—destroy bacteria or inhibit its growth.

A number of serious, often life-threatening illnesses ranging from gastric ulcers and gastroenteritis to *Salmonella, Helicobacter pylori,* and *E. coli* food poisoning result when harmful bacterial strains are free to attach themselves to stomach and/or intestinal walls and multiply rapidly. Once these bacterial infections are out of control, antibiotics are necessary for treatment.

Antibiotics made from cultures of microorganisms or artificially produced in a laboratory, while helpful in killing harmful bacteria, also have a downside. Rash, fever, bronchial tube spasms, inflamed blood vessels, kidney and ear problems, stomach upset, vomiting, diarrhea, fatigue, and insomnia are common side effects of antibiotics. A new problem—the resistance of harmful bacteria to antibiotics—is the result of antibiotic overuse. This overuse has allowed for the development of mutant bacterial strains that are neither destroyed nor inhibited by standard antibiotics. Finally, it is very important to realize that in addition to killing harmful microorganisms, these lab-produced antibiotics also kill essential friendly bacteria. Medical warnings, however, do not mention these serious side effects.

What you may not know is that your friendly bacteria are capable of naturally protecting you against harmful organisms and their devastating effects.

ANTIBACTERIAL, ANTIBIOTIC, AND ANTIMICROBIAL POWERS OF FRIENDLY BACTERIA

Certain strains of friendly bacteria produce powerful antibiotics, all produce acids, and some produce hydrogen peroxide (H_2O_2). Some produce all three. All of these substances effectively inhibit harmful bacteria. Understand, these substances do not actually destroy the pathogenic bacteria, rather they inhibit or scare them away, preventing them from hanging around to do their dirty deeds. The harmful bacteria run from the area, leaving a clean field behind them. This inhibiting action is better than actually destroying the harmful bacteria, which would leave behind toxic debris. Eventually, in order to defend itself from extinction, this remaining bacteria will be forced to mutate. As much as one-third of the dry weight of fecal matter is made of excreted bacteria—harmful, beneficial, and neutral—that your first line of defense has effectively "inhibited" and sent running away.

Unlike lab-produced drugs, the natural antibiotics and other substances made by your beneficial bacteria target harmful bacteria without causing you any uncomfortable and/or dangerous side effects. Researchers E.M. Mikolajcik and I.Y. Hamdan of the U.S. Department of Food Science and Nutrition in Columbus, Ohio extracted acidolin, one of the natural antibiotics, from *L. acidophilus*. Their paper entitled, "Lactobacillus acidophilus II, Antimicrobial Agents," was published in the *Cultured Dairy Products Journal* in late 1975. They reported that the acidolin, "a yellow viscous" liquid, was stable in long-term storage and very active against a wide range of organisms. It did not, however, attack helpful lactic acid bacteria. In addition, acidolin was found to be nontoxic to human tissue cells in culture.

The following Table 7.1, lists a number of beneficial bacteria found in the gastrointestinal tract, and the natural antibiotics they produce.

Table 7.1 Antibiotics Produced by Beneficial Bacteria

BACTERIA	TYPE	SOURCE	ANTIBIOTIC(s) PRODUCED
Bifidobacterium bifidum	Resident.	Bifido-enriched milk; supplements.	Bifidin.
Lactobacillus acidophilus	Resident.	Acidophilus-enriched milk; supplements.	Acidolin, Acidophilin, Lactobacillin, Lactocidin.
Lactobacillus brevis	Transient.	Milk, kefir, cheese, sauerkraut.	Lactobrevin.
Lactobacillus bulgaricus	Transient.	Yogurt, cheese, supplements.	Bulgarican.
Streptococcus lactis	Transient.	Raw milk, raw milk products, cheese, cottage cheese, cultured buttermilk.	Nisin.

Drs. K.M. Shahani and R.C. Chandan were one of the first to successfully isolate the antibiotics they named bulgarican (from the *L. bulgaricus* super strain DDS-14) and acidophilin (from the *L. acidophilus* super strain DDS-1). In 1979, the *Journal of Dairy Science* published the results of their work in an article entitled, "Nutritional and Healthful Aspects of Cultured and Culture-Containing Dairy Products." The researchers concluded that both of these natural antibiotics are "exceedingly active against a wide variety of . . . organisms, which included pathogens and nonpathogens."

TESTING NATURAL ANTIBIOTICS

Once an active agent has been identified and isolated from a substance, it is then tested for strength and efficacy. There are two scientifically accepted ways to establish the worth of a natural substance or drug. The first is to test it under controlled conditions in the lab and, the second, once it has met all safety standards, is to test it on a living entity. If a test is labeled *in vitro*, it was conducted in an artificial environment, such as a test tube or petri dish. If the study is labeled *in vivo* (think "alive"), it was conducted within a living organism, either a lab animal or a human being.

In Vitro Tests

In the laboratory, the scientist begins by growing disease-causing microbes in a petri dish. Once the microbes are growing, the next step is to add the substance to be tested. After a period of time, the area that has been cleared of pathogens by the substance being tested is measured. This area is called the *zone of inhibition*. Clearly, the larger the zone, the more effective the inhibiting substance.

In a 1977 *in vitro* study, Drs. S.E. Gilliland and M.L. Speck confirmed that acidophilin not only fights *Salmonella typhimurium*, but the harmful *S. aureus* and *Clostridium perfringens* bacteria as well. In some instances, specific super strains of *L. acidophilus* showed up to a 98.2 percent zone of inhibition, which means the pathogenic bacteria were frantic to escape and tried to get as far away as possible.

Even though they may be refrigerated, many prepared foods, such as tuna, potato, and macaroni salads made with egg-based mayonnaise, are often contaminated with large numbers of harmful bacteria. Ground beef is another common source of trouble. Dangerous strains of *Staphylococcus, Pseudomonas, Salmonella,* and *Achromobacter*, which actually accelerate food spoilage, can be extremely harmful, even life-threatening, when ingested.

L. bulgaricus is one of the primary organisms that protects yogurt from spoiling. In 1984, Drs. N.M. Abdel-bar and N.D. Harris studied the use of *L. bulgaricus* to protect food against bacterial contamination and subsequent spoilage. Their paper, "Inhibitory Effect of *Lactobacillus bulgaricus* on Psychotrophic Bacteria in Associative Cultures and in Refrigerated Foods," was published in the *Journal of Food Protection*. This study showed that high concentrations of *L. bulgaricus* (between 1.4 million and 5.7 million live organisms per milliliter of concentrate) completely prevented growth of the harmful organisms tested.

The researchers theorized that the combination of acid and hydrogen peroxide (H_2O_2), produced by a strain of *L. bulgaricus,* is what protected the test concentrations against pathogenic microbes. Ground beef is a prime candidate for the protection provided by this friendly bacterial strain. The dangers of *E. coli* contamination of ground beef are widespread. Cooking burgers until they are well-done is strongly advised to kill the harmful bacteria. Even the Meat Association (reluctantly) cautions that meat should be cooked to an internal temperature of 170°F to insure that all harmful bacteria are destroyed. If we can protect our beef with *L. bulgaricus* compounds, we may be able to reduce *E. coli* contamination and eliminate the need for irradiation.

When tested against a number of dangerous microorganisms commonly found in food, acidophilin and bulgarican (extracted from specific super strains) proved to be effective inhibitors of these harmful bacteria. Results were measured by the zone of inhibition.

Table 7.2 is adapted from a paper by G. V. Reddy, K.M. Shahani, B.A.Friend, and R.C. Chandon, entitled, "Natural Antibiotic Activity of *Lactobacillus Acidophilus* and *Bulgaricus*," published in the May, 1983 issue of *Cultured Dairy Products Journal*. This table shows the inhibitory activities of two strains of *L. bulgaricus* and one strain of *L. acidophilus* on a number of pathogenic organisms.

**Table 7.2 Inhibitory Activities of *L. bulgaricus* and
L. acidophilus Strains**

TEST ORGANISMS	*L. BULGARICUS* DDS-13	*L. BULGARICUS* DDS-14	*L. ACIDOPHILUS* DDS-1
Bacillus subtilis	—	++++	+++
Escherichia coli	—	+++	++
Proteus vulgaris	—	+++	++
Pseudomonas aeruginosa	—	+++	++
Pseudomonas fluorescens	—	+++	++
Sarcina lutea	—	++++	+++
Serratia marcescens	—	+++	++
Staphylococcus aureus	—	++++	++
Streptococcus lactis	+/—	+++	++

++++	Very strong inhibition of test culture (zone of inhibition 9–12 mm)
+++	Strong inhibition (zone 5–8 mm)
++	Moderate inhibition (zone 3–4 mm)
+	Weak inhibition (zone 1–2 mm)
—	No inhibition
+/—	Doubtful

In other studies in which the inhibitory activity of bifidobacteria was tested against some of the same dangerous bacteria presented in Table 7.2, the results were almost as impressive. The antibacterial action of bifidobacteria is believed to be due to their production of powerful organic acids, including lactic, acetic, and formic acids. It is known that acetic acid exerts a strong effect on the pathogens *Shigella* and *Salmonella*.

Obviousiy, different strains of bifidobacteria produce different acids of varying intensities. For example, when tests were conducted in 1987, the *B. bifidum* strain designated 1452 was considered the strongest. Today we know that the super strain, Malyoth, is even more powerful.

Table 7.3, taken from Anand, Srinivasan, and Rao's 1984 work entitled, "Antibacterial Activity Associated with *Bifidobacterium Bifidum*," shows the results of the tests in which the *B. bifidum* 1452 strain was used against a number of toxic bacteria. In one test, the bacteria was cultured on nonfat milk, while the other was cultured on broth. As you can see, bifidobacteria—like all members of the *Lactobacillus* family—prefer milk.

In his 1984 paper, "The Role of Bifidobacteria in Enteric Infection," published in *Bifidobacteria Microflora* 5, Dr. R. Ninkaya tested the effects of bifidobacteria on *shigella* bacteria taken from patients suffering with dysentery. First, he took some healthy cells from the intestinal lining of human volunteers and grew them in a culturing medi-

Table 7.3 Effect of *B. bifidum* 1452 on Pathogenic Bacteria

Pathogenic Bacteria	Zone of Inhibition of *B. bifidum* 1452, cultured on nonfat milk	Zone of Inhibition of *B. bifidum* 1452, cultured on broth
Escherichia coli	20 mm	16 mm
Bacillus cereus	22 mm	16 mm
Salmonella typhosa	12 mm	8 mm
Shigella dysenteriae	11 mm	not tested
Micrococcus flavus	25 mm	18 mm
Staphylococcus aureus	23 mm	14 mm
Pseudomonas fluorescens	18 mm	11 mm

um. Next, he set out to learn how much damage *Shigella* bacteria would produce on the unprotected cells, and, more importantly, how much damage could be prevented when the cells were protected by various concentrations of friendly bacteria. In four different phases, Dr. Ninkaya showed that bifidobacteria provided a very real shield against infection.

When *Shigella* was added to the unprotected human cells, approximately 12 percent of the cells became infected. Had this occurred within a living human being, this person would be suffering from dysentery accompanied by severe stomach and abdominal cramps.

When *Shigella* and bifidobacteria were added to the culture at the same time, only 2 percent of the cells became infected. This would probably qualify as a minor episode, possibly characterized by a mild stomachache and abdominal cramps.

When the cells were protected with bifidobacteria for two hours before *Shigella* bacteria were introduced, only 1.6 percent of the cells became infected. This shows that a human protected by vibrant and viable colonies of bifidobacteria is able to shrug off the harmful effects of *Shigella*.

In the fourth phase of his studies, Dr. Ninkaya protected the cells with bifidobacteria, waited for two hours, and washed them clean. Only then did he introduce the *Shigella* bacteria. Even after the cells had seemingly been stripped of the protective bifidobacteria, only 4.4 percent became infected. This is a prime example of the supernatant's protective action, even after the beneficial bacteria have been removed.

It is clear that bifidobacteria protect against *Shigella* very effectively. The most protection was achieved when the bifidobacteria were present and on the job before the disease-causing microorganism was introduced. Consider this a word to the wise. If you have colonies of friendly bacteria in your gastrointestinal tract, chances are you will be less likely to suffer the effects of harmful bacteria.

In Vivo Tests

After the *in vitro* tests have been satisfactorily completed, the next step is to test the substance *in vivo* with lab animals. If the safety of the substance is assured, only then is it tested on humans. The scientifically accepted testing method is to select a number of people and divide them into two groups. One group is given the substance, while the other group, known as the control group, is given a placebo—an inert substance that can neither help nor harm. None of the test subjects knows if he or she is receiving a placebo or the actual test substance. This is called a "double-blind" test.

At the end of a set period of time, the benefits (or lack of) are evaluated in both groups. Ideally, the group given the substance will show positive results, while the control group will not. When evaluating the control group, scientists must take into account what is called the placebo effect—a false sense of improvement. When some people take a placebo that they believe is a medication that will help them, their bodies respond in kind and they actually feel better. In other words, sometimes the mind fools the body into thinking that the "medicine" is a sure cure, causing the symptoms to lessen or vanish.

A number of studies involving the *in vivo* testing of beneficial bacteria in the gastrointestinal tract has shown positive results in the war against harmful microorganisms. Their presence in the urinary and vaginal tracts has proven to be effective, as well.

In the Gastrointestinal Tract

The following studies concentrate on the antibiotic action of beneficial bacteria against harmful microorganisms in the gastrointestinal tract. All are double-blind *in vivo* studies involving real people.

Swedish researchers at the Karolinska Institute have concentrated their studies on the antibiotic properties of a specific strain of acidophilus. One investigation centered on cases of food poisoning by *Salmonella* bacteria. Its goal was to determine if the time the victims harbored the *Salmonella* bacteria was reduced by taking *Lactobacillus acidophilus*. It was. Each day, half of the infected patients in the study were given sixteen ounces (two cups) of acidophilus milk containing 6 billion organisms per milliliter, or around three thousand billion viable bacteria. Compared to the subjects of the control group—who were not given acidophilus milk, but were instead treated with standard medical antibiotics—the patients helped by the friendly bacteria had a much shorter period of sickness before the infection was resolved. In other words, the subjects who drank the acidophilus milk recovered from the *Salmonella* food poisoning faster than the subjects on standard antibiotics.

In another study, sixteen Polish children with dysentery caused by *Salmonella* and fifteen with dysentery caused by *Shigella* were given the bacteria-enriched acidophilus milk. After the initial treatment, seven children with *Salmonella* and ten with *Shigella* were free of symptoms. As the treatment went on, all of the children were cleared of their infections.

A six-month study of the preventive properties of cultured milk products involved 1,000 Japanese soldiers. Half of the soldiers received yakult, a Japanese fermented milk drink cultured with Lactobacillus casei, shirota strain. At the end of the six-month period, not one of the 500 soldiers drinking the yakult had contracted dysentery. On the other hand, fifty-five of the soldiers in the control group who were not given yakult had dysentery, and another fifty were found to be infected with Salmonella or Shigella, even though they showed no overt symptoms.

Cancer patients who are treated with chemotherapy drugs quickly show disturbances in their gastrointestinal tracts. Their intestinal flora becomes densely populated with both anaerobic and aerobic harmful bacteria, including *Klebsiella, Citrobacter,* and *Proteus vulgaris. Bacteroides* also increase significantly, and the troublesome yeast fungus *Candida albicans* takes advantage of the opportunity to spread out and take over new territories.

When the bacterial balance in the intestines shifts from friend to foe in this way, the overgrowth of harmful microbes makes it an ideal testing ground for studies using bifidobacteria and lactobacilli. In one Japanese study, medical scientists concentrated their research on fifty-six leukemia patients who were undergoing chemotherapy. They tested blood and urine samples for toxins created by pathogenic bacteria. They also isolated, identified, and estimated the numbers of intestinal bacteria and classified the levels of candida proliferation in the fifty-six patients.

Yeast overgrowth proved to be a serious problem. Four patients registered 100 million candida organisms per gram of intestinal contents; six patients registered 10 million organisms per gram; and four patients showed 1 million organisms per gram. Three patients at similar levels of candida overgrowth were kept separate as part of the control groups.

While the control groups did not receive supplemental friendly bacteria, the test groups of patients received milk that was enriched with high levels of bifidobacteria and acidophilus. Each milliliter of milk contained 20 million organisms (half bifido and half acidophilus); the patients drank 200 milliliters of the bacteria-enriched milk daily for three months.

Dramatic improvements were noted in the patients who drank the enriched milk. At the end of the study, not one patient who received the friendly bacteria supplements showed more than 1 million microorganisms of candida per gram in their stool samples. No changes were reported in the control groups.

In the Urinary Tract

You may be surprised to learn that most urinary tract infections are caused by bowel bacteria—often *E. coli, Proteus, Klebsiella,* or an *Enterobacter* species—coming from the intestinal tract. Such infections are seldom seated in the bladder, but usually in the urethra, the narrow tube that carries urine from the bladder out of the body.

Symptoms of urinary tract infections include the need to urinate frequently and burning, painful urinations. If the infection is severe, there may be blood and/or pus in the urine. Urinary tract infections are more common in women than in men. In fact, men may suffer from a urinary tract infection and not know it, as they seldom have overt symptoms. The standard medical treatment includes antibacterial drugs, pain relievers, and urinary antiseptic drugs.

In England, a Liverpool-based urologist, Dr. R.M. Jameson, believes in a different approach for treating urinary tract infections. In 1976, he authored a paper entitled, "The Prevention of Recurrent Urinary Tract Infection in Women," published in *The Practitioner.* His study focused on female patients whose frequent urinations were coupled with pain and burning. Dr. Jameson placed the women on a high-fiber, sugar-free diet. This intake reduction of refined carbohydrates improved both the chemistry of their urinary tract and their bowel flora. To assist in the rapid recolonization of the gastrointestinal tract with friendly bacteria, Dr. Jameson had his patients take acidophilus supplements, and suggested yogurt be a part of their daily diets. He writes, "It cannot be emphasized too strongly that this dietary regimen is designed to produce, not just symptomatic relief, but a lifelong cure."

In their 1987 paper published in *FEMS Microbiology Reviews* entitled, "The Therapeutic Role of Dietary Lactobacilli and Lactobacillus Fermented Dairy Products," Drs. C.F. Fernandes, K.M. Shahani, and M.A. Amer pointed to bacteria such as *E. coli, Klebsiella, Proteus,* and *Pseudomonas,* and the overgrowth of *Candida albicans* as the major sources of both urinary and vaginal tract infections. These researchers state, "The normal urethral, vaginal, and cervical flora of healthy females can competitively block the attachment of pathogenic bacteria to the surfaces of cells in women with and without a history of urinary tract infections." They point out that the activity of the lactobacilli stops invading bacteria from adhering to the urethral and vaginal surfaces, and stress that this ability can be used to both protect against infection and to restore the normal bacterial balance once infection has taken place.

In the Vaginal Tract

In 1892, a German obstetrician by the name of Albert Doderlein identified and described the characteristics of what came to be known as the Doderlein bacillus. The name is still used today, but Dr. Doderlein's bacteria is now better known as *L. acidophilus*. Bacteria, friendly and otherwise, are reclassified all the time as more of their characteristics are identified.

Today we know that *L. acidophilus* is a normal and protective inhabitant of the vaginal tract, but in the 1920s, researcher Dr. R. Schröder was the first to recognize that the pH and bacterial count of his patients' vaginal secretions provided an indication of that region's health. After he completed his original studies, he was able to categorize his nonpregnant patients by three grades.

His grade-one patients, which constituted 40 percent of his subjects, had vaginal secretions that were decidedly acidic. These secretions registered nearly exclusive amounts of beneficial Doderlein bacillus (*L. acidophilus*) and very few pathogens. His grade-two patients, which included about 18 percent of the women tested, showed a combination of Doderlein, pathogenic, and neutral bacteria. Dr. Schröder's grade-three patients, constituting around 42 percent of his study subjects, had high-alkaline vaginal secretions. These secretions harbored a vast number of pathogens, including diptheroids, *Streptococci*, and *Micrococci*. Very few beneficial Doderlein bacteria were present. All of these grade-three patients were experiencing vaginitis.

Vaginitis, or inflammation of the vaginal tract lining, is characterized by a burning and/or itching sensation and a foul-smelling discharge. Although there are many prescription and over-the-counter preparations designed to treat vaginitis today, they come with decided drawbacks. First of all, many treatments provide symptomatic relief, but seldom effect a true cure. This is especially true if the condition is due to a yeast infection. According to a 1996 study conducted by the manufacturers of Diflucan, a product designed to treat vaginitis, 85 percent of American women will suffer from nonspecific vaginitis at least once in their lifetime. Many of these women will experience recurring infections again and again. No matter what the root cause of the trouble may be, yeast or bacteria, the condition is likely to return again and again unless steps are taken to normalize the region's friendly bacterial count.

In his *Textbook of Natural Medicine*, Paul Reilly, N.D., addresses the use of acidophilus in treating vaginitis. He writes, "Whenever there is a disturbance of the normal vaginal flora, re-establishment of these organisms is important. This may be accomplished by the insertion of live lactobacillus culture yogurt. . ."

Another study showing the effectiveness of treating various forms of vaginitis with nothing but pure cultures of *L. acidophilus* was conducted by B.C. Butler and J.W. Beakley in 1960. Their paper entitled "Bacterial Flora in Vaginitis," reported in issue 79 of the *American Journal of Obstetrics & Gynecology*, described the study. When acidophilus supplements were introduced into the vaginal area of the study subjects, the pathogenic bacteria (commonly *Staphylococcus*, *Streptococcus*, and *Diplococcus*) were largely replaced with the beneficial Doderlein bacillus. The pH balance of the area shifted from an alkaline pH level between 5 and 6 to a more acidic pH level of 4. The symptoms of vaginitis were quickly relieved, and, with the maintenance of healthy acidophilus supplements, did not recur.

Table 7.4, adapted from the study by Butler and Beakley, shows the effects of *L. acidophilus* (Doderlein bacillus) on different types of vaginitis.

Table 7.4 Effects of *L. acidophilus* on Vaginitis

TYPE OF VAGINITIS	NUMBER OF SUBJECTS	CURE RATE	SYMPTOMATIC CURE RATE	FAILURE RATE	RECURRENCE RATE
Nonspecific	19	95%	5%	0	0
Monilia	25	88%	12%	0	0
Trichomonas	8	87%	0	13%	25%
Trichomonas and monilia	6	100%	0	0	0

The September–October 1990 issue of *Reviews of Infectious Diseases* published an article entitled, "Emerging Role of Lactobacilli in the Control and Maintenance of the Vaginal Bacterial Microflora," authored by researchers of Wayne State University School of Medicine (Detroit). This study emphasizes the role that vaginal lactobacilli play in controlling the vaginal microflora and maintaining a normal state. According to the report, "Lactobacilli possess many antagonistic properties and produce many metabolites that may be important in maintaining dominance in the vagina." As explanation, the study cites . . . "growth inhibition of *Gardnerella* and other anaerobic bacteria to acid production by lactobacilli. . . competition for adherence [to vaginal walls]. . . hydrogen peroxide production. . . [and] broad-spectrum antimicrobial agents."

Other studies using recolonizing bacteria confirm that this simple approach to treating vaginitis with special strains of friendly bacteria really works. *L. acidophilus* and, to a lesser degree, *L. bulgaricus* cultures are both successful in restoring acidity and repopulating the vagina when used as a treatment for vaginitis.

What is most important is that effective treatment is dependent on the right strain of the right bacteria. A 1991 University of Washington School of Medicine study, published in *The Journal of Infectious Diseases*, authored by S.J. Klebanoff, S.L. Hillier, D.A. Eschenbach, and A.M. Waltersdorph entitled, "Control of the Microbial Flora of the Vagina by H_2O_2-Generating Lactobacilli," confirms that the best bacteria for normalizing vaginal microflora is a lactobacillus strain that produces hydrogen peroxide (H_2O_2). This work is consistent with other findings and confirms that hydrogen peroxide-generating lactobacilli are present normally in the vagina of most women, but are most often absent from women with bacterial vaginal infections. This study (in which this particular lactobacilli are referred to as "LB") showed that, "LB at high concentration was toxic to *Gardnerella vaginalis* (the predominant organism in the vagina of women with BV [bacterial vaginosis]," and also stated that, "LB alone as low concentrations was toxic to *Bacteroides bivius* through the formation of H_2O_2. . . These findings suggest that LB may contribute to the control of the vaginal flora. . ."

Because research into this problem has been repeated many times, it has been concluded that when there are few (or no) lactobacilli present in the vagina—even though the patient has no symptoms—it can be assumed that bacterial vaginitis will soon erupt, even when no pathogenic bacteria can be located.

A 1990 Canadian study entitled, "Hydrogen Peroxide Production by *Lactobacillus* Species: Correlation with Susceptibility to the Spermicidal Compound Nonoxynol-9" had a different slant. Nonoxynol-9 is the active component of many spermicidal preparations. This study documented the disturbing fact that the vaginal flora of spermicide users can be depleted of hydrogen peroxide-producing lactobacilli, which can increase the susceptibility to urogenital infection. The report states, "Women using diaphragms and spermicides as a means of contraception are at an increased risk of acquiring urinary tract infections and bacterial vaginosis. In addition, *E. coli* is recovered twice as frequently from the vaginas of diaphragm users . . . than from women using other forms of contraception. It has been suggested that this is due, in part, to spermicidal compounds altering the vaginal flora. . . This study shows a good correlation between the sensitivity of lactobacilli to the action of nonoxynol-9 and production of H_2O_2. The lactobacilli, which are extremely susceptible to low concentrations of nonoxynol-9, would be expected to be killed in spermicide users thus removing the potentially protective H_2O_2 producers. The nonoxynol-9-resistant lactobacilli would remain but might not afford protection against urogenital infections because they do not produce H_2O_2." Women using a diaphragm or a spermicide are well advised to enlist the services of the right strain of supplemental hydrogen peroxide-producing friendly bacteria.

Perhaps you have heard that using yogurt as a douche is an effective way to treat vaginitis. It is and it isn't. First of all, supermarket yogurt won't do. Only properly cultured, pure yogurt containing live bacteria cultures of *L. bulgaricus* and *S. thermophilus* can help ease the itch. Second, these friendly transient bacteria are helpful, but they aren't the best choice. It is *L. acidophilus,* the colonizer, that really works.

However, simply eating acidophilus-enriched yogurt daily has been documented as a viable treatment for vaginitis. A study entitled, "Ingestion of Yogurt Containing *Lactobacillus acidophilus* as Prophylaxis for Candidal Vaginitis," published in the March 1992 issue of *The Annals of Internal Medicine,* showed that eating eight ounces of acidophilus-enriched yogurt daily for six months decreased both candidal colonization and vaginal infections.

This information was based on a study of thirteen women who suffered regular bouts of vaginitis. Its purpose was to see if the regular ingestion of yogurt with acidophilus would decrease the number of episodes of vaginal candidiasis. The team of doctors involved explained, "The current therapies [for vaginitis] are often inadequate and many patients fail treatment; however, reports on systemic prophylaxis have been promising. . . All patients who crossed over from 'no yogurt' to yogurt reported subjective relief."

An interesting note—the high-quality commercial yogurt used in the above study contained hydrogen peroxide producing *L. acidophilus* and *L. bulgaricus*. Six months after the conclusion of this study, however, the manufacturer reformulated the product. Why? Although the exact reasons were never made public, one can only speculate that the product was changed to one that took less time to produce, and was, therefore, commercially more profitable.

When the vaginal secretions of healthy women with no gynecological disorders are tested, all are found to have healthy resident colonies of acidophilus. I believe the reason recolonizing the vaginal area with *L. acidophilus* isn't used universally is either because there's no way for the giant drug companies to make a profit on a natural remedy, or because of a lack of awareness of the method, since it is not taught in medical schools in the United States.

CONCLUSION

This chapter has described the antibiotic power of the friendly bacteria. While I certainly don't recommend that you start eating undercooked hamburgers or eggs that may be contaminated with *Salmonella*, it is nice to know that as long as you have living, thriving colonies of beneficial intestinal bacteria, they will help protect you against the dangers of these contaminants. It's a good idea to augment your diet with probiotic supplements to insure that your friendly bacteria are always deployed in full strength. Health begins within your gastrointestinal tract.

8

The Antiviral Activity of Friendly Bacteria

A virus is a tiny organism that can grow only within the cells of another organism. When your doctor says you have a viral infection, he or she means that you have a disease caused by one of the 200-plus harmful viruses that science has identified so far.

Although some viruses are harmless, others can cause some of the most dangerous diseases we know. Notoriously difficult to treat, common viruses include the adenovirus, which affects the lungs, stomach, and intestines; the enterovirus, which mainly affects the intestinal tract; the rhinovirus, which causes about 40 percent of respiratory diseases; influenza (the flu), which is characterized by general discomfort, but also can be deadly; the poliovirus, which can cause paralysis; and the herpesvirus. Herpesvirus includes many related viruses, such as simplex 1 and 2, which affects the skin and genitals; varicella-zoster, the cause of chicken pox and the source of shingles; Epstein-Barr virus, the cause of mononucleosis and extreme fatigue; cytomegalovirus, which can cause blindness and is very serious in newborns and those with impaired immune systems; and the Human immunodeficiency virus (HIV), which leads to acquired immune deficiency syndrome (AIDS), a systematic destroyer of the immune system.

Viruses can enter your body in many ways. Some, like HIV and herpes (HSV-2), are sexually transmitted. Intravenous drug users who share needles are at great risk of contracting HIV and other serious infections. Some viruses can sneak into the body through cuts in the skin, while others are inhaled through the lungs, and yet others are ingested with food or water. While you can lessen your chances of getting some viruses (practicing safe sex, for instance), there is no way you can avoid exposure to all of them.

THE HANTAVIRUS—HOW A NEW STRAIN INFILTRATED SOCIETY

New viruses as well as new strains of known viruses are always infiltrating society. You may remember that in 1993, a "new" disease—a previously unknown strain of hantavirus—surfaced in the Navajo nation of New Mexico. The mortality rate in those infected was around 70 percent. What began with flu-like symptoms that affected the respiratory system, ended in death for many—and all within a few days.

Of the 119 people who were eventually infected with this strain of hantavirus, 59 died as the disease attacked their lungs. Before the true cause was discovered, early cases listed the cause of death as "acute respiratory distress syndrome (ARDS) of unknown etiology." One reason why the investigators originally dismissed the possibility of hantavirus is because all previously identified hantaviruses caused kidney problems, not respiratory complications.

Before the cause of this "new disease" was discovered, tribal medicine men and elders, always very close to nature, were consulted by investigators from the Centers for Disease Control (CDC). They noted that the mouse population and pinon nut harvest were unusually large that spring. They also remembered the great epidemics of 1918 and 1936 as times when both the mouse population and the nut harvest had been very high. This was the clue the CDC needed to send the investigators in the right direction.

In a lucky coincidence, an ongoing survey of the local rodent population by the University of New Mexico had already documented a ten-fold increase in deer mice in the area. This study quickly confirmed the observations of the Navajo elders and led to the determination that the common deer mouse carried the hantavirus. When humans came in contact with viral-contaminated urine or feces of the infected mice, they contracted the disease.

The world first took notice of hantavirus when more than 2,500 American soldiers fighting in Korea fell ill with a mysterious disease.

Of those infected, 121 died of kidney failure. U.S. Army researchers determined that the virus was carried by field mice.

Hantaviruses have also surfaced in Europe and Asia and have eventually made their way around the world, causing chronic kidney problems, ranging from mild to severe. It has been shown that those who come in contact with a hantavirus are ten times more likely to develop serious kidney disease. In the United States, tests run on a number of patients undergoing kidney dialysis revealed that 6.5 percent had been infected with a slow-growing hantavirus at some time in the past. It is believed that many hundreds of cases of unexplained ARDS and kidney disease may eventually be traced to infection by one of the hantaviruses.

MEDICAL ANTIVIRAL STRATEGY

Medical science is still seeking effective ways to treat viral diseases. As you know, drugs classified as antibiotics destroy bacteria. However, to date, there is no class of drugs that destroys viruses overall, although scientists are working tirelessly to come up with more effective treatments for all viral conditions, including AIDS.

Although gains have been made in the development of antiviral agents against specific viruses (some strains of herpes and influenza, for example), success in the war against all viruses is elusive. In addition, all antivirals—indeed, all drugs—have side effects. Nonetheless, great strides have been made in the war against viral infections. Consider the almost-complete eradication of poliomyelitis due to the development of the Salk and Sabine vaccines in the mid-1950s. Many childhood viral diseases, including chickenpox, smallpox, measles, and mumps have been all but eliminated thanks to the development of specific vaccines.

So far, it is apparent that the most effective approach to beating a viral invasion is to prevent it from becoming successful once it enters the body. The friendly bacteria can help do just that.

ANTIVIRAL CONTROL FACTORS

Like lab-produced vaccines, the beneficial bacteria living in your gastrointestinal tract help prevent certain viral invasions from becoming serious threats. Although science has not yet pinpointed the exact mechanism by which your friendly bacteria head off viral complications, Emanuel Revici, M.D., founder of the Institute of Applied Biology in New York, believed that the evolutionary hierarchy of the microorganisms offers a clue.

Because viruses are older than bacteria on the evolutionary scale, Dr. Revici theorized that many forms of bacteria had to develop methods of controlling viruses in order to protect themselves as they evolved. Obviously, if all bacteria were at the mercy of all viruses, the bacteria—both good and bad—would have died out long ago.

The internal control factors that friendly bacteria have at their disposal to work against viruses are not fully understood. However, we do know that lactobacilli produce large amounts of lactic and other acids, and viruses are not comfortable in an acidic environment. We also know that the friendly bacteria have the ability to raise the temperature in their territory, and viruses have difficulty coping with high temperature levels. Friendly bacteria also synthesize certain byproducts, such as essential fatty acids, that viruses cannot tolerate.

Dr. Revici's work centered on the use of "good" bacteria to control undesirable viral activity. He determined that special strains of specific bacteria, like lactobacilli, secrete viricidal compounds that actually kill viruses. One of the most important of these viricidal compounds is hydrogen peroxide (H_2O_2). Studies have confirmed that the secretions of these friendly bacteria help them fight the viruses that invade their territory.

ANTIVIRAL ACTION OF LACTOBACILLI

In Chapter 7, you saw the powers of acidolin—the natural antibiotic extracted from *L. acidophilus*—against bacterial infections. Although lab-produced antibiotics have no effect on viruses, acidolin has both antibiotic and antiviral properties.

In their paper, "Acidolin: An Antibiotic Produced by *Lactobacillus acidophilus*," published in *The Journal of Antibiotics,* I.Y. Hamdan and E.M. Mikolajcik explained their 1974 study. After culturing colonies of the polio virus and vaccinia (cowpox) virus, they added various concentrations of acidolin. They confirmed that a dilution of 1 part acidolin to 80 parts inert liquid produced "complete disintegration" of both the polio and vaccinia cells. Disintegration of the vaccinia virus was accomplished at a concentration of 1 part acidolin to 160 parts liquid, showing that vaccinia was even more sensitive to the acidolin than the polio virus.

The researchers also noted that with increased concentration of acidolin, the culture medium increased in acidity. At a very mild acid reading of pH 6.5 to 6.8 (pH 7 is neutral), no disintegration was observed. However, when more acidolin was added, the medium went from pH 6.5, at a concentration of 1 part acidolin in 320, to an extremely acid reading of pH 3.6, when the concentration of acidolin was 1 part in 80. This concentration proved to be the undoing of both the polio and vaccinia viruses. The potential viral troublemakers were turned off, deactivated, and terminated.

On Herpesvirus

In 1983, the *E.E.N.T. Digest* published a paper by D.J. Weekes entitled, "Management of Herpes Simplex With a Virostatic Bacterial Agent." Dr. Weekes reported on case studies from his files involving patients struggling with the aftereffects of taking broad-spectrum antibiotics for long periods of time. These patients suffered from diarrhea, a common consequence when antibiotics cause a die-off of beneficial intestinal bacteria. They also suffered from severe herpes simplex lesions in the mouth, as well as some types of nonviral mouth ulcers that often accompany the herpesvirus.

Dr. Weekes treated these patients with active *L. acidophilus* and *L. bulgaricus* tablets. The patients were instructed to dissolve four 25 mg acidophilus and/or bulgaricus tablets in their mouth with milk four times daily. All of the patients improved; both the diarrhea and mouth lesions disappeared.

After this success, Dr. Weekes began treating other forms of the herpesvirus by the same method. In one study, he used the same treatment shown above on sixty-four patients with vaginal herpes (herpes simplex labialis), ninety-seven with mouth lesions (aphthous stomatitis), thirteen with ulcers of the cornea (dendritic ulceration), and six with genital herpes (herpes progenitalis). All of the patients with genital herpes were cured. For vaginal herpes, the beneficial bacteria achieved a 95 percent success rate; thirty-seven of sixty-four patients were cured, and twenty-four were much improved. For most, the benefits came within three days. Only three patients showed no change. The success rate in those patients with herpes sores in their mouths was around 80 percent; forty of ninety-seven patients were cured, thirty-seven were much improved, and twenty showed no change. Improvements were noted within twenty-four hours, and the lesions disappeared within four days for the 80 percent who were helped. Most people are unaware that herpes can infect the cornea of the eye, but it can. The success rate here was 46 percent, with six patients cured out of the thirteen treated.

Dr. Weekes reports that only three patients who took the friendly bacteria noticed any side effects. All three experienced mild gastrointestinal reactions, probably due to the normalizing effect of the bacteria in the gastrointestinal tract.

This is another instance in which acidic pH levels are perhaps part of the cure. Dr. Weekes noticed that dissolving strain-specific lactobacillus tablets in the mouth raised levels of the acidic salivary enzyme *phosphatase*, and he theorized that the high degree of acidity promoted by the friendly bacteria might be a factor in deactivating the viruses.

In his paper, Dr. Weekes added one caveat. He wrote, "No claim is made that herpetic or aphthous [mouth] lesions will not recur after cessation of therapy with viable lactobacilli. However, results indicate that individual attacks may be cured, improved, or suppressed by prompt use of the preparation. Used early enough, it will actually abort the clinical aspects of the viral process and will speed healing when used at any stage."

Dr. Weekes also remarked on the preventive effects of acidophilus on herpes-induced mouth sores. He described a patient who developed mouth ulcers whenever she drank orange juice, which she dearly loved. As long as she took acidophilus daily, the orange juice did not bother her. Deciding on her own that she was permanently cured, she stopped taking the supplement and continued drinking orange juice. The herpes lesions returned. When she went back on the acidophilus supplement, the mouth sores stopped.

In Baltimore, Drs. L. Rapoport and W.I. Levine also reported outstanding results in treating herpes-induced lesions and mouth ulcers with a combination of acidophilus and bulgaricus. Their paper, "Treatment of Oral Ulceration with Lactobacillus Tablets," was published in 1965 in Issue 20 of *Oral Surgery, Oral Medicine, and Oral Pathology*. Patients were instructed to take from two to four tablets daily for two or three days, depending on how severely they were infected. The body size and weight of each patient was also factored in when deciding on the prescribed number of doses.

To evaluate the results, the physicians established strict criteria. Unless the patient reported "unequivocal relief of pain within forty-eight hours, the results were considered negative." That's a pretty tough schedule for any medication to meet, but the physicians were not disappointed. Of the forty patients treated with lactobacilli, thirty-eight reported complete relief of pain within forty-eight hours and thirty-six reported disappearance of the lesions within five days. No side effects were reported.

On HIV Virus and AIDS

Recent research has indicated that friendly bacteria may affect the transmission of the HIV virus that causes AIDS. The heterosexual transmission of HIV is occurring with increasing frequency. In the transmission of the HIV virus between a man and a woman, it has been determined that the virus often survives the local defense mechanisms of the body. It's important to note that passing on the virus can go both ways; by this I mean that an infected woman can transmit the virus to a man, just as easily as an HIV-positive man can infect a woman.

In 1991, the Department of Medicine of the University of Washington set up a controlled *in vitro* study to address the problem of heterosexual transmission of the HIV virus. In a paper entitled "Viricidal Effect of *Lactobacillus acidophilus* on Human Immunodeficiency Virus Type 1: Possible Role in Heterosexual Transmission," S.J. Klebanoff and R.W. Coombs reported that H_2O_2-generating lactobacteria, a type of bacteria that is normally present in human vaginal secretions, may help defeat the HIV virus. They wrote, "H_2O_2-generating *Lactobacillus acidophilus* (LB+) is present in the vagina of most normal women, and peroxidase has been detected in vaginal fluid. LB+ at high concentration is viricidal to HIV-1 and, at levels where LB+ is ineffective alone, the addition of peroxidase . . . and a halide restore viricidal activity. LB+ can be replaced by H_2O_2 (peroxide), but not by non- H_2O_2-producing LB. . . . The survival of HIV in the female genital tract and thus the likelihood of transmission may be influenced by the activity of the LB+-peroxidase-halide system in the vagina."

Therefore, "Normal individuals, or persons with sexually transmitted vaginal disease in whom vaginal H_2O_2-producing lactobacilli are few or absent, may thus be at greater risk of infection and, as a corollary, may benefit from vaginal colonization with H_2O_2-generating lactobacilli." To put it simply, this study found that large numbers of lactobacilli that produce hydrogen-positive peroxide in the vagina tract, inhibit sexual transmission of the HIV virus.

It is important to note that the researchers said, "the likelihood of transmission may be influenced." Remember, this was an *in vitro* study in which the results came from observing the activity of the organisms in a petri dish, not in human beings. So, although this is encouraging news from the world of science, further studies are needed.

In his work entitled, "Possible Treatment of AIDS patients with Live Lactobacteria," published in 1988 in *Medical Hypotheses*, Dr. F. Tihole of Ljubljana, Yugoslavia, points to the "enhancement of antimicrobial resistance and immunomodulatory action and anabolic effect caused by the consumption of live lactobacteria as a dietary adjunct . . . as sufficient reasons to test lactobacterial preparations in patients with AIDS." Dr. Tihole's paper reviews the many benefits of the friendly bacteria and concludes by saying, "Given that these physiological and therapeutic effects of lactobacteria lead to improved antimicrobial resistance, it would seem well worth testing this treatment on AIDS patients as well."

CONCLUSION

Unless you are willing to live in a plastic bubble and have no contact whatsoever with the outside world, there is no way to avoid coming in contact with viruses. They are in the air we breathe, the water we drink, and the food we eat. Unfortunately, I can't promise you that taking probiotic supplements of friendly bacteria will give you complete immunity against all viruses. However, there is clear evidence showing that selected strains of lactobacilli can protect you against exposure to nasty herpes and flu viruses. And, as you have seen, the friendly bacteria can help relieve symptoms of these viruses if you do become infected.

9

The Anti-Cancer Capabilities of Friendly Bacteria

Your body is made up of around 75 trillion cells. Through an orderly process called mitosis, or cell division, new cells develop from pre-existing ones. This is how the human body grows. Unlike normal cells, cancer cells do not follow this orderly growth pattern; they do not play by the rules. Unreceptive to the normal signal to stop reproducing, they multiply uncontrollably and eventually form a lump, or tumor. Tumor growth eventually interferes with the ability of the different body structures to perform their appointed functions. The result is illness or death.

Most cancer types, of which there are more than 150, have different causes, different symptoms, and vary in aggressiveness. Most types fall under four general categories:

1. Carcinomas, which affect the skin, glands, and internal organs.
2. Sarcomas, which affect muscles and bones.
3. Lymphomas, which affect the lymphatic system.
4. Leukemias, which are cancers of blood-forming tissue.

In all of these categories, with the exception of leukemia, cancerous cells multiply to form malignant (cancerous) tumors. Not all tumors, however, are malignant. Benign growths, unlike malignant ones, are usually encapsulated within a membrane, and, although they may grow larger, they do not spread to other areas of the body. The word benign literally means "harmless."

In its early stages, cancer is very difficult to detect. When examined under a microscope, a young cancer cell looks very much like the healthy cell in which it originated. However, once this cell begins to multiply wildly, duplicating itself into a malignant lump, the cancerous cells can no longer be recognized as offspring of the original healthy cell.

Many cancers spread (metastasize) to other parts of the body by releasing cancer cells into the bloodstream or lymphatic system. These cells are then carried to other areas of the body, often far from the original site, where they begin reproducing.

Although we don't know exactly why some cells become cancerous, we do know that certain factors increase the odds of certain cancer types. Environmental factors and diet are the two major causes, although genetic predisposition and stress are also believed to play a part.

Carcinogens—substances that can cause the growth of cancer—are lurking everywhere. You can't escape them all, even if you try. Environmental carcinogens include any of the many natural or manufactured substances that can cause cancer. They include chemical agents, physical agents, and certain hormones and viruses. Some

Cancer's Warning Signs

Knowing cancer's early warning signs can save your life. The symptoms listed below have been associated with various types of cancer. If you experience one or more of these symptoms, it does not necessarily mean that you have cancer (many of these symptoms can be caused by other, less serious illnesses). You should, however, contact you doctor or other professional health care provider for an evaluation.

1. An unexplained change in bowel or bladder habits.
2. A sore that doesn't heal.
3. Unusual bleeding or discharge.
4. A thickening or lump (in the breast or elsewhere).
5. Indigestion or difficulty in swallowing.
6. An obvious change in a wart or mole.
7. A persistent, nagging cough and continued hoarseness.

common carcinogenic substances include arsenic, asbestos, uranium, vinyl chloride, radiation, ultraviolet rays, x-rays, vehicle emissions, and various substances derived from coal tar.

REDUCING YOUR CANCER RISKS

Although it is impossible to avoid all of the risk factors of developing cancer, be aware that sound lifestyle choices can reduce your odds tremendously. Many of the factors that add to your risk of developing cancer are under your personal control.

Using tobacco, in any form, increases the possibility of lung, mouth, esophageal, and—surprisingly—pancreatic cancer. Exposure to second-hand smoke from cigarettes, pipes, and cigars is dangerous as well. Regular consumption of alcohol can lead to mouth, throat, and liver cancer. Exposure to sunlight is implicated in skin cancer. Poor diets—those lacking in essential vitamins, minerals, and nutrients—have been implicated in stomach and colon cancers. Let's take a closer look at these dietary decisions.

CANCER AND DIET

Since the 1940s, researchers observed that diet influences the progress of cancer. Scientists have long known that tumors induced in lab animals grow faster when the animal's diet is high in fat. Too much fat in the diet—especially saturated animal fat—not only promotes high cholesterol levels, but also inhibits the action of important immune system cells.

As mentioned earlier, one of the primary reasons for the uncontrolled proliferation of cancer cells is due to carcinogens. And they are everywhere. Take nitrosamines, for example. These carcinogenic substances are produced in the body from the nitrites and nitrates used in the curing of ham and other luncheon meats, bacon, sausage, kielbasa, and hot dogs. On one hand, nitrates and nitrites prevent the formation of deadly botulism spores. On the other hand, these chemicals produce carcinogenic nitrosamines, which increase the risk of esophageal, stomach, and colon cancer. Believe it or not, there is some good news here. Healthy colonies of friendly bacteria have the ability to neutralize nitrites before they can be transformed into dangerous nitrosamines.

Remember, a diet high in animal fats and fried foods has been shown to be a contributor to stomach, colon, breast, prostate, and pancreatic cancers. When the diet is unbalanced in favor of an excess of animal protein, putrefaction in the gastrointestinal tract is common. Ecological changes in the bowel lead to a loss of friendly bacteria and a rise of harmful ones, with a subsequent increase in highly toxic and cancer-causing substances.

To further illustrate the importance of diet, consider the following results of one study performed on a group of laboratory rats. Half of the rats were fed an all-grain diet, while the other half was given a diet rich in beef. All of the rats were given the cancer-causing agent DMH (1, 2, dimethylhydrazine). Of the grain-fed rats, only 31 percent developed cancer of the colon, while 83 percent of the beef-fed rats developed the same.

The protective effects of the friendly bacteria were also confirmed in this study. When the beef-fed rats were given DMH (the cancer-causing substance) along with *L. acidophilus*, only around half as many, 40 percent, of the group developed cancer after twenty weeks. However, by the end of the study (thirty-six weeks), 77 percent of the rats had colon cancer. Although these acidophilus-fed rats initially showed a resistance to cancer, the beef diet eventually broke down this resistance.

The implications of this study are clear. Even with the friendly bacteria on guard, which certainly helps in the fight against illness, probiotic supplementation should be only part of your complete program for good health. A healthy diet is also necessary for total protection.

Harmful bacteria in the gastrointestinal tract can be involved in certain chemical changes that can result in the formation of carcinogens. When the balance shifts in favor of potentially dangerous bacteria, they gain strength and go to work, producing certain enzymes that are able to transform some usually harmless chemical byproducts of digestion, known as procarcinogens, into full-fledged carcinogenic factors. Yet another reason why it's important for your resident friendly bacteria to be strong.

THE CANCER-FIGHTING FRIENDLY BACTERIA

When *Lactobacillus acidophilus* bacteria are present in sufficient strength, many of the potentially dangerous digestive enzymes produced by harmful bacteria (such as b-glucuronidase, b-glucosidase, and nitro-reductase) are not able to cause problems. Studies show these enzymes are slowed dramatically by your friendly bacterial army.

In their 1987 report, "The Therapeutic Role of Dietary Lactobacilli and Lactobacillic Fermented Dairy Products," published in *FEMS Microbiology Reviews,* Drs. C.F. Fernandes, K.M. Shahani, and M.A. Amer listed three cancer-fighting capabilities displayed by the friendly bacteria.

First, certain super strains of your friendly bacteria eliminate pro-carcinogenic substances before they can turn carcinogenic. Among these are the nitrites mentioned earlier. Before the substances can be converted into cancer-causing carcinogens in your intestinal tract, specific strains of *L. acidophilus* step in and neutralize them. Even better, the best of the friendly bacteria super strains have the ability to metabolize any procarcinogens that escape and convert them back into noncarcinogenic substances.

Second, beneficial bacteria are capable of altering certain enzymes (such as b-glucuronidase and nitro-reductase) that turn procarcinogens into carcinogenic agents. The "bad" bacteria that secrete these destructive enzymes include *Clostridium* and certain *Bacteroides,* among others. Obviously, the more dangerous enzymes that are present in your gastrointestinal tract, the greater your risk of harboring cancer-causing substances. The ability of active super strains of *L. acidophilus* bacteria to neutralize these harmful enzymes is one of their most important contributions to cancer prevention.

Third, by a mechanism that is not fully understood, lactobacilli have the mysterious ability to directly suppress some tumor activity. Jean M. Antoine cites a wealth of studies in his December 1989 report entitled, "Validation of Health Attributes of Yogurt." In the section on cancer, Dr. Antoine says, "Studies on experimental cancers induced in animals demonstrated that yogurt strains were able to slow down the evolution of various cancers." The section concludes with this statement, "It looks like yogurt strains in the gut could reduce the quantity or quality of toxins produced during the digestion, absorption and colic fermentation of our food."

In yet another paper entitled, "The Role of Diet in the Causation and Prevention of Cancer," published in 1989, Barry R. Goldin of Tufts University School of Medicine (Boston), discusses the same subject. Presenting data drawn from six different studies, Goldin shows that fermented dairy products are capable of slowing tumor induction and growth. Table 9.1, below, is an adaptation of the study results.

Based on his research, Dr. Goldin calls diet a major factor in the development of cancer. He states, "Statistical analyses of incidence data indicate that approximately 35 percent of all cancers are diet related." What you eat does make a difference in your health, and it seems apparent that the anticarcinogenic properties of the friendly bacteria play an important role in the internal fight against cancer.

A BACTERIAL BOOST TO YOUR IMMUNE SYSTEM

Although the friendly bacteria are your first line of defense against disease, your immune system has the heavy responsibility of keeping you well. Your immune system identifies foreign intruders that have gotten past the friendly bacteria, and produces antibodies to conquer

Table 9.1 Inhibiting Action of Fermented Dairy Products on Tumor Growth

AGENT	INHIBITING ACTION
Yogurt	25–35 percent inhibition of transplantable cancer-causing Ehrlich cells in mice.
Fermented colostrum with DDS-1	16–41 percent inhibition of cancerous ascites cells in mice.
Cultured milk with *L. acidophilus* DDS-1	Inhibited tumor proliferation by 16–41 percent in mice.
Cultured milk with *L. acidophilus, L. bulgaricus,* and *L. bulgaricus* plus *S. thermophilus*	Inhibition of cancerous ascites cells in mice.
Milk fermented with *L. acidophilus* and *thermophilus*	Decreased mortality in rats challenged with the colon carcinogen DMH (cancer-causing agent).
Sour milk	Inhibition of DMH-induced tumors in rats.
Scandinavian ropy sour milk (lang fill or villi)	50–75 percent inhibition of sarcoma cells injected in mice.

these invaders. In addition, scavenger cells called macrophages gobble up invaders, mutant cells, metabolic trash, and the harmful chemicals that enter your body through the water you drink, the food you eat, and the air you breathe.

Once, the main functions of your immune system were the production of antibodies against disease; the destruction of dangerous bacterial, fungal, and viral invaders; and the elimination of mutant cells that have the potential to turn cancerous. Now, the immune system's workload is further complicated by the need to cleanse the body of the increasing number of extraneous pollutants and contaminants found in the environment and the food chain. Overloaded with work, the immune system needs all the help it can get from your friendly bacteria. How? When disease-causing aliens are able to permeate the intestinal walls and enter the bloodstream, the immune system must spring into action. As long as strong colonies of friendly bacteria line the intestinal tract in full force, these harmful microorganisms will not be able to get through, thus lightening the already heavy workload of the immune system. As you will see, several *in vitro* and *in vivo* studies illustrating the ability of the friendly bacteria to boost immune function have been performed.

Laboratory Study

In order to determine how well *L. acidophilus* and *S. thermophilus* work to boost the immune system, in 1987, Argentinean researchers performed a study using laboratory mice. In this study, the mice were divided into three main groups. All received their normal ration of mouse chow. Along with their food, the mice in Group One received live bacteria—some were fed *L. acidophilus* or *S. thermophilus*, while the others were injected with these same live bacteria. The mice in Group Two received deactivated (dead) bacteria—some were fed the bacteria with their food, others were injected with it. The mice in Group Three—the control group—were denied bacteria in any form.

By the second day, it was clear that the mice given live *L. acidophilus*, either by mouth or injection, fared the best. Compared to the control mice, macrophage activity was increased between three and four times, a clear indication of enhanced immune system activity. Mice receiving certain strains of *S. thermophilus* showed some increased activity, but this transient "yogurt" bacteria did not measure up to acidophilus. The mice receiving deactivated (dead) bacteria registered at the same levels as the mice who received no bacteria at all.

The researchers concluded, "Since activation in the body of macrophages is important in suppressing tumor growth, immunostimulation by the oral route might well be a new approach by stimulating the specific and non-specific immunity of the host."

Other Studies

Several studies in humans have also shown the value of friendly bacteria in raising immune system function and helping to lower the risk of cancer.

Dr. D.J. Henteges and associates at the University of Missouri were involved in a study on the effects of eating red meat. The results of this study were presented in a paper entitled, "Effect of High-Beef Diet on the Fecal Bacterial Flora of Humans," published in *Cancer Research* in 1977. In the first month of the study, ten volunteers went on what was termed a "control" diet, during which they ate a small amount of beef—eighty grams (three ounces)—once a day. In the second month, beef was eliminated entirely. During the third month, the volunteers ate a very high-meat diet consisting of 800 grams (a little over ten-and-a-half ounces) of meat every day. For the fourth and final month, the subjects went back on the control diet and consumed only eighty grams of meat daily.

Tests revealed that during all four stages, the concentration of friendly bifidobacteria in the large intestine remained at a level of 10 billion organisms per gram of feces. However, the harmful *Bacteroides* underwent some population shifts. For the first month, on the control diet, and during the second "meatless" month, the *Bacteroid* levels remained at a low 10 billion organisms per gram. During the high-meat month, the level rose dramatically to 100 billion organisms per gram. They remained at the same high levels during the final month, even though the low-meat diet was back in effect.

Lactobacilli dropped from a high of 10 million organisms per gram for the first two months to a low of only 1 million organisms per gram during the third month of the high-meat intake. When the meat intake dropped again in the final month, the lactobacilli levels returned to around 10 million.

The research team concluded that these dietary changes made only a marginal impact on the intestinal flora, but I disagree. Only the desirable bifidobacteria of the large intestines were relatively unaffected, but the best bacterial friends we have in the small intestine—the lactobacilli—were greatly reduced during the high-meat month. The potentially dangerous *Bacteroides* made the highest gains, and these levels did not fall during the final month. In addition, all of the volunteers continued to eat a high-fat diet of around eighty grams whether they were eating meat or not. The amount of fat you consume makes a great deal of difference to the friendly bacteria.

In a paper entitled, "Nutritional and Therapeutic Aspects of Lactobacilli," published in the *Journal of Applied Nutrition,* Drs. Khem Shahani and B.A. Friend reported on their 1984 study. In this study, they attempted to show that friendly bacteria alter the production of the dangerous enzymes that produce active carcinogens from procarcinogens. To find out what effect *L. acidophilus* milk had against these enzymes, they tested changes in the microflora of two groups of geriatric patients whose diets had been supplemented with either acidophilus milk or plain milk.

Drinking plain milk did not affect the microflora at all. But drinking acidophilus milk dramatically reduced the activity of two enzymes—b-glucuronidase and b-glucosidase—that produce carcinogenic changes in procarcinogens. The researchers also discovered that even when the acidophilus milk supplementation stopped, the colonies of *L. acidophilus* bacteria that had been established during the trial period flourished for some time and continued their protective effects. This study proved that simply supplementing the diet with acidophilus milk succeeded in reducing levels of putrefaction and decreasing the formation of cancer-causing materials in the gastrointestinal tract.

In 1980, the *National Cancer Institute* published a paper entitled, "Effect of Diet and *Lactobacillus acidophilus* Supplements on Human Fecal Bacterial Enzymes," written by Dr. B. R. Goldin and associates. Knowing that vegetarians produce far fewer of the dangerous enzymes than meat-eaters, these scientists set out to determine if changing the diet of meat-eaters and/or supplementing their diets with lactobacilli would result in a lower production of the offensive enzymes.

First, they increased the fiber content of subjects' meals for one month, then extended it to two months. The added fiber showed no effect on the levels of three dangerous enzymes (b-glucuronidase, nitro-reductase, and azo-reductase). However, the subjects did register a reduction in a fourth undesirable enzyme (7-a-dehydroxilase).

Next, for the same length of time, the red meat was removed from the subjects' diets, although white meat was still allowed. This dietary change had no effect at all on the levels of dangerous enzymes; they remained high. Obviously, red meat, as well as animal proteins and fats, lead to the putrefaction that gives the dangerous enzymes free rein.

However, when the subjects were allowed to eat the meats of their choice, but took *Lactobacillus acidophilus* supplements, there was a marked reduction in the levels of b-glucuronidase and nitro-reductase. When supplementation stopped, the levels of the dangerous enzymes increased again.

Studies on Cancer Patients

Dr. Ivan Bogdanov of Sofia, Bulgaria, is a world-renowned authority on intestinal bacteria who has been researching the benefits of *L. bulgaricus* for many years. The following information is derived from two of Dr. Bogdanov's best-known works: his authoritative 1982 monograph, *Observations on the Therapeutic Effect of the Anti-Cancer Preparation from Lactobacillus bulgaricus (LB-51) Tested on 100 Oncological Patients*, published by the Laboratory for the Research and Production of Biologically Active Substances (Sofia, Bulgaria), and a paper issued jointly by Drs. Bogdanov and P.G. Dalev entitled, "Antitumor Glycopeptides from *Lactobacillus bulgaricus* Cell Wall," published in *FEBS Letters* in 1975.

Dr. Bogdanov has been working with his favorite friendly bacteria—*Lactobacillus bulgaricus*—for almost half a century. It was back in 1951 that he isolated the antibiotic produced by *L. bulgaricus* LB-51. In 1956, he discovered that this same super strain produces a cancer-fighting agent that kills tumor cells without harming surrounding cells. When you realize that all existing chemotherapeutic agents depress the immune system, cause serious side effects, and are terribly toxic to the human body, you can appreciate the importance of his findings. The extracts from LB-51 do not cause nasty side effects or allergic reactions, and they actually stimulate the immune system into greater efforts against a tumor.

Working in Bulgaria, Dr. Bogdanov and his colleagues identified and isolated three different chemical agents from *L. bulgaricus* that were used effectively against cancerous sarcomas and ascitic tumors. The extracts were named "blastolysins" and they were found to be effective, specifically against cancerous tumors induced in mice. However, tumor cells exposed to the bulgaricus extracts in a petri dish were unaffected. The obvious conclusion was that, in Dr. Bogdanov's words, "Blastolysin activates the animal's immunological mechanisms." What could be better? A substance that improves the immune response against cancerous tumors is a great victory in the ongoing war against one of the world's major causes of death.

Dr. Bogdanov's team demonstrated that it was actually a component of the cell wall of *L. bulgaricus,* called a peptoglycan, that carried the anti-tumor properties. Peptoglycans are present in the cells walls of some, but not all, lactobacilli.

In their 1984 study, Drs. B.A. Friend and K.M. Shahani confirmed this effect in a paper entitled, "Nutritional and Therapeutic Aspects of Lactobacilli," published in the *Journal of Applied Nutrition.* In addition, they reported that similar anti-cancer activity occurs when extracts of *L. acidophilus, L. casei,* and *L. helveticus* are used in treating sarcomas in mice. Dr. Shahani emphasized that *L. acidophilus* super strain DDS-1 produced the strongest anti-tumor activity.

Other researchers have been eager to build on Dr. Bogdanov's work as well. In his paper, "Lactic Acid Bacteria and Human Health," published in the *Annals of Medicine* 22:37–41, 1990, Dr. Sherwood L. Gorbach cited Dr. Bogdanov's pioneering findings on three glycopeptides that show activity against sarcoma-180 and solid Ehrlich ascites tumors. Dr. Gorbach's work demonstrated that oral supplementation with viable *L. acidophilus* super strains initiated a decline in the enzymes that cause procarcinogens to become active carcinogens in the large bowel. Dr. Gorbach states, "These studies show that the addition of this strain of *Lactobacillus* to the diet can delay colon tumor formation. . . . In a more recent study from our laboratory, we have shown that oral *L. acidophilus* supplementation to the diet in rats lowers the amount of carcinogenic amines excreted in the feces. . . This corroborates our earlier findings that lactobacilli suppress the metabolic activity of the colonic microflora and in this manner may reduce the formation of carcinogens in the large intestine."

Originally, Dr. Bogdanov used the bulgaricus extract intravenously, but subsequent findings, such as those cited above, show that there are advantages to taking it by mouth. Absorption is rapid and effectiveness seems to be enhanced by oral treatment. And volunteers taking the substance report that it produces no harmful side effects.

In his monograph, Dr. Bogdanov remarked on "the stimulatory effect of the preparation on the regeneration processes in the organism." In other words, the patients taking the bulgaricus extract were not only more responsive to treatment, but the side effects of radiation and chemotherapy were less destructive. He found that even patients in the advanced stages of cancer, who had received radiation and/or chemotherapy were suffering through the side effects of these treatments, tolerated the bulgaricus extract very well.

In 1967 in Sofia, Bulgaria, Dr. Bogdanov ran clinical trials involving the *bulgaricus* LB-51 extract (called Anabol), on human patients with various cancers. Although megadoses of up to thirty and forty grams of Anabol showed actual tumor disintegration, they also produced a toxic reaction. Bits of the tumor had to be cleaned up by the body's detoxification systems, including the liver, the gastrointestinal tract, and immune system cells. That's why a low, steady, continuous oral dose was determined to be best, especially for the seriously weakened patients selected for this study.

The average daily dose of Anabol was between ten and fifteen grams. At least three months of treatment were necessary to achieve what Dr. Bogdanov calls the "anti-tumor effect." For most of the patients in this study, the minimum length of treatment was six months, with many patients continuing its use for between two and four years. The longest continuing treatment lasted nine years. Although these time periods may seem very long, remember that many of the patients treated with Anabol in this study were considered to be terminal. The doctors had tried everything at their disposal and, except for pain relief, had nothing left to offer. In Dr. Bogdanov's study, the L. *bulgaricus* extracts scored a tremendous victory over cancer.

The study subjects were separated into three groups. Group A was comprised primarily of seriously ill cancer patients in the terminal stages of the disease. Those in Group B suffered from severe side effects brought on by simultaneous chemotherapy and radiation treatments, including unremitting nausea, vomiting, pervasive weakness, and hair loss. The Group C subjects included those whose bone marrow had been seriously damaged by radiation and chemotherapy. This side effect is very dangerous, as infection-fighting white blood cells are produced in the bone marrow. When the bone marrow can no longer produce white blood cells, the immune system cannot operate efficiently.

Among the forty-five severely ill patients in Group A there were cases of pancreatic, thyroid, bladder, laryngeal, breast, stomach, lung, rectal, uterine, ovarian, and brain cancer. Other cancers in this group included malignant melanoma, multiple melanoma, sarcoma, and Hodgkin's disease. all of the conventional treatments that medical science had to offer had been tried without success. The patients had been sent home from the hospital with strong pain killers and not much else.

What follows is the case history of one of the subjects in Group A. It is typical of many of the other patients. This information is taken from Dr. Bogdanov's 1982 monograph, referenced above.

S.K.B., male, age 57.
Diagnosis: Multiple myeloma, cachexia, uremia, coma.
Histological diagnosis: Plasmocytoma.

May, 1968
Diagnosis at admission:
Chronic nephritis. Intolerable bone pains and severe cachexia develop, with atrophy of muscle mass (the patient cannot lift his hand). X-ray shows multiple overlapping myeloma foci in bones. Diagnosis confirmed by needle biopsy. Gradually becoming somnolent; in the course of one week, uremic coma developed.

Results of laboratory analysis immediately before initiation of Anabol treatment: Hb 44, urea 160 mg percent, ESR 140–160 mm/hr.

7/12/1968
Anabol treatment began as only therapy, patient moribund, general condition improved rapidly in the course of one week. Patient recovered consciousness. Pains decreased.

In two weeks, voice was restored. No spontaneous pains. Opiates discontinued. Urea 44 mg percent, ESR 34–63 mm/hr.

10/3/1968
General condition improved constantly. Muscles of chest and arms gradually recuperated.

12/15/1968
Five months after initiation of Anabol treatment, general condition
very good. The body muscles are almost completely recovered except for
legs, which remind us of the recent severe cachectic state of the patient.

7/1/1969
In good general health. No clinical evidence of disease. Walks alone,
using only a cane. Discharged from clinic. Lives in village. Takes care
of himself, able to carry out work without strenuous physical exercise.

1/1/1970
Complete remission without evidence of recurrence continued for sev-
enteen months.

This case history was typical of the subjects in Group A. In the
majority of patients treated with oral Anabol as their only therapy,
most showed a wide range of improvement. Some had complete
regression of their cancers, and no harmful side effects were reported.
Even after six years of using Anabol, the benefits continued for most
of the patients in this group.

The patients in Group B were those experiencing severe side effects
due to chemotherapy and radiation treatments. All of the subjects in this
group were treated with Anabol, and all showed marked improvement.
As the toxic effects of their previous treatments were eased, many
became strong enough to tolerate going back on chemotherapy.

The Group C patients whose bone marrow had been seriously
damaged by radiation and chemotherapy also responded well to the
Anabol. Most showed rapid therapeutic effects, even in the most
severe cases of subjects with very low white blood cell counts.

After actively treating patients with LB-51 extracts for many years,
Dr. Bogdanov summarized his findings by saying that the preparation
has "a *therapeutic* effect in incurable cancer patients in whom all other
methods have failed, and a *protective* effect against the harmful effects
of other forms of cancer treatment, ensuring a maximum use of their
potential for tumor destruction. It also has a *therapeutic* effect where
there has been severe radiation and chemotherapy damage, and the
benefits are seen within a few days."

Countless case histories in Dr. Bogdanov's files confirm the effects
of the *L. bulgaricus* LB-51 preparation. It not only eases the side effects

of conventional cancer treatments like chemotherapy and radiation, including bone marrow damage, but even terminal cancer patients respond quickly, gain strength, and grow well with this simple, non-toxic treatment.

You're probably asking the same question Dr. Bogdanov asks, "Why not use it before the terminal stage is reached?" I have no answer, except to remark that in the west (the United States in particular) clinical studies from Eastern Europe and the Former Soviet Union are routinely dismissed. It is unfortunate that more research following Dr. Bogdanov's model was not duplicated in the United States.

However, it may interest you to know that the Japanese are so impressed with Dr. Bogdanov's findings that a Japanese consortium is funding the construction of what is to be called the "The L.B. Center" in Sofia, Bulgaria. (Just in case you didn't catch it, L.B. stands for *Lactobacillus bulgaricus*.) Japanese researchers and medical doctors will be working with their Bogdanov-inspired Bulgarian counterparts. I'm looking forward with great interest to the additional solid documentation on the impressive effects of L.B. that I'm sure will be forthcoming from this group of dedicated scientists.

CONCLUSION

Through scientific research, you have seen how your friendly bacteria can reduce the threat of potential cancer-causing agents in your body, increase your body's immune function, and neutralize dangerous enzymes that have the ability to turn procarcinogens into active carcinogens.

I wish I could tell you that simply eating a bowl of real yogurt every day will prevent cancer. Unfortunately, this is not all it takes. So many factors are involved in the development of this disease—viruses, environmental pollutants, genetic predisposition—that there is no single solution. However, some cancer risk factors are under your control, especially diet. As you have seen, simply lowering the amount of fat and red meat you eat can measurably lower your risk of developing cancer. And the friendly bacteria have been shown to reduce levels of dangerous, carcinogen-forming enzymes in your gastrointestinal tract, as well as boost the function of your immune system. Supplementing your diet with probiotics, in addition to healthy dietary choices, is one way to help lower your risk of getting cancer.

10

Choosing the Right Probiotics

*I*t is possible to arm your body with the kind of friendly super bacteria that can go up against such dangerous microorganisms as *E. coli, Salmonella,* and *Candida albicans* and win, but you must know how to select the proper probiotics. Just as not all strains of bacteria are the same, not all probiotics are the same. The effectiveness of a probiotic supplement depends on what it contains, how it is prepared and processed, and how it is packaged. This chapter is designed to give you some important guidelines to follow when selecting probiotic supplements.

THE RIGHT BACTERIA

Probiotic supplements of resident bacteria should be taken daily to maintain the health and well being of your friendly bacteria. When their numbers have been depleted for any reason—illness, antibiotic therapy, candida overgrowth, and so on—you need to take therapeutic doses of bacteria in the billions to restore your beneficial colonies to vibrant health.

One type of bacteria cannot substitute for another. The most important friendly colonizing bacteria for continued good health and the integrity of your gastrointestinal tract are *Lactobacillus acidophilus,* found mainly in your small intestines, and *Bifidobacteria bifidum,* common to your large intestines. These friendly bacteria not only produce and liberate numerous beneficial substances, including vitamins, amino acids, antibiotics, and other antimicrobial substances, but they are necessary for maximizing the absorption and utilization of nutrients.

Beneficial transient bacteria play a different role. These travelers don't set up colonies, but they do a lot of good as they pass through the body. Much as a fertilizer helps plants grow, transient bacteria help resident bacteria to flourish. The friendly "yogurt" bacteria, *Lactobacillus bulgaricus* and *Streptococcus thermophilus*, are the best known, most active, and most beneficial of these transient bacteria. It's important for you to include both the right residential and transient bacteria as part of an effective supplementation program.

THE RIGHT STRAIN

In order to produce superior quality probiotics, it is necessary to start with the right strain of each of the beneficial bacteria. If the strain is weak, the end product won't do you much good.

As explained in Chapter 3, some bacterial strains within the same family are much better (or much worse) than others. For example, almost all *E. coli* strains are harmless, but a few strains—like the lethal 0157:H7—are so powerful that they can be deadly. On the other hand, almost all beneficial bacterial strains are harmless. A very few super strains are very powerful and absolutely lethal to some deadly bacteria, including *E. coli* 0157. Other strains are so weak they are virtually useless. It is imperative for you to choose wisely.

When shopping for probiotics, always look for the most powerful strains of each species—ones that have retained their beneficial supernatants (see The All-Important Supernatant on page 115). These super strains are presented in the following discussions.

Lactobacillus acidophilus

There are approximately 200 different known strains of *L. acidophilus*, and they are definitely not created equal. Of these strains, only thirteen have good antibiotic qualities.

Dr. Khem Shahani warns, "All acidophilus products available commercially are not prepared alike. The name on the bottle does not mean anything to the consumer if the bottle does not contain the right acidophilus strain. Many strains cannot even survive human gut fluid and bile salts." The DDS-1 super strain and the dairy-free NAS super adhesion strain are the ones most highly recommended.

The All-Important Supernatant

Friendly bacteria are grown in a culturing medium, usually milk. As the bacteria grow, they transform the milk into a new substance that is known as the supernatant. This supernatant growth base contains beneficial metabolic byproducts that are helpful to both you and the bacteria. These include antimicrobial compounds (such as hydrogen peroxide and acidophilin), vitamins, enzymes, cellular building blocks, antioxidants, and immunostimulants.

Beware probiotic products that have been processed using centrifugation or ultrafiltration (see pages 122–123). These methods, which are the easiest and least expensive form of processing, remove the invaluable supernatant, resulting in an inferior product. The full-culture processing method is necessary to keep the bacteria and its all-important supernatant together.

L. acidophilus DDS-1 Super Strain

Studied extensively by Dr. Shahani and his associates at the University of Nebraska, the *L. acidophilus* DDS-1 super strain has been shown to be the most effective against the widest number of pathogens. Among its many capabilities, the DDS-1 strain produces extremely effective natural antibiotic substances that can inhibit eleven known disease-causing bacteria.

When the thirteen acidophilus strains were tested against nine nasty organisms—*Bacillus subtilis, Serratia marcescens, Proteus vulgaris, Pseudomonas fluorescens, Pseudomonas aeruginosa, Escherichia coli, Sarcina lutea, Streptococcus lactis,* and *Staphylococcus aureus*—DDS-1 was the clear winner. It was found to have, in Dr. Shahani's words, "very strong inhibition against six test organisms and strong inhibition against three test organisms." Another strain of acidophilus—DDS-8—tested very strongly against three of these organisms, strongly against one, moderately against four, and weakly against one.

The DDS-1 strain also has been proven to inhibit yeast infections, improve chronic constipation and/or diarrhea (by normalizing the gastrointestinal tract), aid in nutrient uptake (especially of calcium), and prevent food poisoning by targeting the harmful bacteria. It has strong antimicrobial activity against a wide range of common pathogens and shows good assimilation of "bad" cholesterol. Be aware, however, that DDS-1 demonstrated its uncommonly strong antibiotic properties only when it was cultured in a milk base.

The only way to retain all the important properties of the DDS-1 super strain in a dairy-free formula is to fool these good guys into thinking their cozy "nest" is milk based. If you need a dairy-free formula, be sure the bacteria were carefully nurtured in a vegetable base that mimics the exact carbohydrate/protein ratio found in milk.

I have found the best *L. acidophilus* DDS-1 and NAS super strains to be hydrogen peroxide positive, which means they provide added activity against harmful bacteria. Prominent United States researcher Dr. Sharon Hillier, as well as a number of others, has confirmed the importance of such a feature.

The DDS-1 hydrogen peroxide-positive super strain is highly recommended for overall daily maintenance. When the small intestine and upper gastrointestinal tract are under attack from such problems as candida infestation, increased amounts of this super strain can provide the extra support needed to fight the harmful overgrowth. This strain also can be helpful for those with food, chemical, and environmental sensitivities; microbial or fungal overgrowth syndromes; chronic immune suppression; dysbiosis (toxic bowel and/or toxic liver); nutrient malabsorption; B-complex deficiencies; inflammation of the small intestine or stomach; diarrhea and/or constipation; and high cholesterol levels. It helps break down bacterial enzymes and/or potential cancer-causing agents. In addition, it can give support during and after the use of antibiotics, steroids, chemotherapy, bulking agents, intestinal cleansing programs, and antimicrobial herbs such as echinacea, goldenseal, and garlic.

When selecting a probiotic acidophilus supplement, be very suspicious if the manufacturer doesn't specify the strain. A "something dophilus" product is most likely produced with an inexpensive strain that won't do you any good at all. When judging acidophilus products, remember that the DDS-1 strain is the one you want.

DDS stands for the University of Nebraska's *Department of Dairy Science*, where this strain was discovered. Be aware, however, that there are products out there carrying a misleading "DDS" designation that have nothing to do with the true DDS-1 strain. Even worse, some probiotic labelers have adopted DDS as a trademark for marketing purposes. Unfortunately, these products do not include the true DDS-1 organism identified in the original research, and the organisms are not produced according to published specifications.

Know that all DDS-1 strains are not created equal. Only probiotics produced from the true DDS-1 culture—identified by its DNA "fingerprint"—and grown according to the exact specifications that insure maximization of its health-giving properties can deliver the benefits promised by all the studies mentioned in this book.

In conclusion, when choosing *L. acidophilus*, to select a DDS-1 super strain formula that provides 2 billion living bacteria through a guaranteed expiration date. This super strain comes in milk-based powders and capsules, as well as in dairy-free formulas. And remember to select a product that retains its supernatant growth medium (see page 115).

L. acidophilus NAS Super Adhesion Strain (Dairy-Free)

The NAS "sticker" strain adheres readily to the intestinal lining without requiring the presence of calcium ions, making it the perfect dairy-free acidophilus product. The product you want provides 2 billion living *L. acidophilus* of the NAS super strain in a certified organic culture base of modified garbanzo bean (chick pea) extract. And make sure you select a product that retains the original supernatant growth medium (see The All-Important Supernatant on page 115). The uses for specially cultured dairy-free acidophilus are the same as for the milk-grown DDS-1 super strain, described above.

Bifidobacteria

Bifidobacteria are (or should be) the major inhabitants of the large intestine. They compete fiercely for both nutrients and attachment sites along the intestinal walls, preventing invasions of pathogenic bacteria, including yeasts. Bifidobacteria are prodigious producers of acids that lower the pH, thus increasing the acidity of the region. This function makes the area unattractive to harmful bacteria that prefer an alkaline environment. When bifidobacteria are present in force, invaders cannot survive. In addition, bifidobacteria inhibit the bad bacteria that alter nitrates (ingested in food or water) into nitrites, which are potential cancer-causing agents. They also aid in the production of B-complex vitamins and assist in the dietary management of the liver.

Although the super strains of the bifidobacteria do all these good things to everyone, an age-specific species is recommended. This means that in addition to having been cultured with a super strain, the probiotic must also be suitable for the age of the individual. For adults, the *B. bifidum* Malyoth strain is best, while infants and young children require the gentler *Bifidobacterium infantis*, preferably the NLS super strain.

Bifidobacteria bifidum Malyoth Super Strain

Bifidum probiotics formulated with the Malyoth super strain are recommended for overall support, large intestine therapy; liver detoxification; food, chemical, and environmental sensitivities; microbial or fungal overgrowth syndromes; chronic immune suppression; dysbiosis (toxic bowel and/or toxic liver); nutrient malabsorption; B-complex deficiencies; inflammation of the large intestine; breakdown of bacterial enzymes and/or potential cancer-causing agents; support during and after the use of antibiotics, steroids, chemotherapy, antimicrobial herbs such as echinacea, goldenseal, and garlic, bulking agents, and intestinal cleansing programs; and diarrhea and/or constipation.

Look for products, capsules, or powder, that provide two billion living *B. bifidum* Malyoth super strain, in either a base of nonfat milk and whey, or a dairy-free organic base of modified garbanzo bean extract. Be sure you choose a brand that retains the original supernatant growth medium (see page 115).

Bifidobacteria infantis NLS Super Strain

If there is a beloved infant in your family, I invite you to review Chapter 5 to understand the importance of giving the youngest among us a good start in life by putting probiotics on the menu. Select a probiotic formula that contains two billion living *B. infantis* NLS super strain, in a base of nonfat milk and whey. Choose a product with a printed expiration date, and one that retains the original supernatant growth medium.

Some babies may be genetically allergic to the casein—a protein found in milk. Unless you know for certain that milk is easily tolerated in your family, do not give a dairy-based product to your infant. (For more information on casein intolerance, see page 41.)

The NLS super strain of bifidobacteria is recommended for overall support of your infant because they stimulate better weight gain through nitrogen retention, especially important for formula-fed infants; assist in the production of B vitamins and the absorption of calcium and other vitamins and minerals; help produce lactase, the enzyme required to break down milk sugar; help prevent a predisposition to allergies; inhibit colonization of the intestine by disease-causing bacteria; and encourage the formation of antibodies against undesirable bacteria and viruses.

B. infantis supplementation is especially important for babies delivered by cesarean section and those who are not breastfed. As well, this supplement is important during and after antibiotic therapy, after immunizations, and when the baby is experiencing an intestinal or digestive disturbance. Whenever there is a dietary change or when traveling, especially to developing countries, *B. infantis* supplementation is suggested.

Babies born vaginally to healthy mothers receive their initial supply of friendly bacteria on their passage through the birth canal. Science can't explain how this phenomenon occurs, but it does. To make sure your child is provided with the right strain of bacteria from birth on, I recommend that pregnant women and nursing mothers augment their usual probiotic supplementation with *B. infantis* as well. Babies delivered by cesarean section are especially in need of probiotic supplementation.

Along with their own personal program of probiotics, pregnant women should take ½ to 1 teaspoon of *B. infantis* NLS super strain powder stirred into unchilled filtered water daily, beginning in the third trimester of pregnancy. While you are nursing your baby, continue taking your own "big three" trinity of probiotics, plus ½ to 1 teaspoon of the NLS super strain powder stirred into unchilled filtered water daily. If your child is a "lazy nurser," try mixing the powder well with a small amount of unchilled filtered water and give it to the baby by dropper. You can also dab a little diluted powder on your nipples to be sure your baby receives the full benefit of this important "infant strain" of friendly bacteria.

Bottle-fed babies should receive ⅛ to ½ teaspoon of NLS super strain powder every day. Just dilute the powder in a little unchilled filtered water and add it to three of your baby's bottles daily. If your child is one who seldom finishes a bottle, give the probiotic by dropper, or use the larger dosage to be sure he or she gets the full benefit.

When the intestinal flora of babies and very young children is disturbed by a decline in bifidobacteria levels, which can be caused by changes in nutrition, a course of antibiotics, or even the necessary inoculations against childhood diseases, the use of supplemental bifidobacteria can assist immeasurably by restoring the correct balance of bacteria in their intestinal tracts.

Lactobacillus bulgaricus

Although *L. bulgaricus* is a transient bacteria—not a colonizer—it is a great help to the resident bacteria that set up colonies in your intestines. The most effective strain is LB-51.

Lactobacillus bulgaricus LB-51 Super Strain

The *L. bulgaricus* LB-51 strain is so powerful it is known as the "supreme strain." Although it is especially "famous" for alleviating digestive problems (including acid reflux) and taming a runaway appetite, everyone can benefit greatly from it. The LB-51 super strain is recommended for overall support of the friendly bacteria, enhanced digestibility of milk products and other proteins, production of natural antibiotic substances, inhibition of undesirable organisms, maximum effectiveness of waste disposal, colon cleansing without disrupting friendly bacteria, and effective immune enhancement.

LB-51 has been extremely well-researched by many recognized scientists, and has proven to be a winner every time. Bulgarian Dr. I.G. Bogdanov and his associates first isolated this strain in 1951. They established that LB-51 synthesizes a natural antibiotic substance that has such a wide spectrum of activity that it has been used successfully for many years by Bulgarian doctors to treat such gastrointestinal disorders as enterocolitis.

A transient bacteria, *L bulgaricus* is most effective in powder or wafer form, not capsule. Be sure the product you select provides 2 billion living *L. bulgaricus* LB-51 super strain, in a base of nonfat milk and whey. Remember, as always, select probiotics that retain the original supernatant growth medium, which provides very special beneficial products of great benefit to you and the friendly bacteria.

CULTURING FRIENDLY BACTERIA

Once the correct super strain has been selected, probiotic products are made very much the same way as real yogurt. These friendly bacteria are grown in what is called a "culturing medium," and milk is the preferred culturing agent. As the bacteria grow, they transform the milk into a totally different substance called the *supernatant*. A very important component of "super" probiotics, the supernatant is filled with a variety of beneficial metabolic byproducts including antimicrobial compounds (hydrogen peroxide, acidophilin) vitamins, enzymes, cellular building blocks, antioxidants, and immunostimulants. But what about those who require dairy-free probiotics? Let's begin by discussing the culturing of these bacteria.

Dairy-Free Probiotics

In lactose-intolerant or lactose-allergic individuals, milk-based products (including some milk-grown probiotics) can cause a host of problems ranging from a "fire" on the tongue, to an outbreak of hives, to severe intestinal distress. Because friendly bacteria produce lactase in response to their own needs, probiotics (even those with a milk-base) often can be used by those who are lactose-intolerant, but not always. In some highly allergic individuals, nondairy-based probiotics are tolerated best. Those who are genetically intolerant to the casein (protein) in milk and milk products must choose nondairy probiotics only. (For additional information on casein intolerance, see the inset on page 41.)

It is possible, even easy, to take friendly bacteria that has been grown in milk and continue to grow it in a dairy-free medium for a few generations. After several generations, the bacteria will "forget" that they are a milk-loving bacteria and will keep right on growing, generation after generation. However, they will also "forget" how to produce lactase—the special byproduct your intestinal tract needs. In other words, later generations of the bacteria that are grown in a medium other than milk will eventually lose their ability to produce lactase, because they no longer need it. They must be grown in a customized vegetarian formula that helps the bacteria produce those indispensable beneficial byproducts that are found in the supernatant.

When shopping for dairy-free probiotics, "let the buyer beware" definitely applies. Many manufacturers have responded to the needs of lactose-intolerant individuals by providing dairy-free probiotic varieties; however, consumers looking for true dairy-free probiotics cannot rely on label information alone. This is because United States government standards allow a little leeway in labeling information, which can be somewhat misleading.

Probiotics may be labeled "dairy-free" and legally still contain a percentage of dairy byproducts (much the same way that an "alcohol-free" wine can legally contain up to 5 percent alcohol). Two of the most common processing methods—centrifuging and ultra-filtration—separate the bacteria from the milk-based supernatant, which is then discarded. By discarding the milk they were grown in, manufacturers can still legally label their probiotic product "dairy-free," even though the bacteria may still have some milk byproducts clinging to them.

This means that the so-called "dairy-free" bacteria processed by centrifuging or ultrafiltration may still contain the legal limit of milk byproducts. But even worse, many centrifuged or ultrafiltrated bacteria are weak and ineffective. They have lost the power and protection of the supernatant. Keep this fact in mind while I tell you how most commercial probiotics are processed.

PROCESSING THE BACTERIA

When a full-grown batch of bacteria is ready to be marketed, manufacturers use different methods to process the product. Centrifuging and ultrafiltration are two popular although inferior methods. Both methods separate and concentrate the bacterial mass, and throw out the invaluable supernatant.

The full-culture production method is the most desirable. It retains the entire bacterial mass including the valuable supernatant. Once processed, all bacteria is then freeze dried (lyophilized).

Centrifugation and Ultrafiltration

When a full-grown batch of bacteria is ready for processing, many manufacturers use the centrifuge method, which is the easiest and least expensive route. It is also the least desirable for a quality product.

The bacteria and supernatant are dumped into a centrifuge, and with the flip of a switch, they are thrown against the sides of the centrifuge with tremendous force. Many of the bacteria end up with ruptured cell walls, while others are killed outright. Bacteria form themselves into chains as they multiply; during the centrifugal process, these chains are broken.

In spite of the damage centrifuging does to beneficial bacteria, it remains a popular processing method because it is easy and cheap. Many manufacturers claim separating the bacteria from its milk base makes it a safe nondairy product. Not true. As explained earlier, the most effective nondairy product is cultivated in a customized vegetarian formula that helps the bacteria produce those indispensable beneficial byproducts in the supernatant. Unfortunately, for many manufacturers, easy and cheap are more important than quality.

With growing public awareness of the damage that centrifugal force can cause to probiotics, some manufacturers have switched to a less-harmful processing method—ultrafiltration. In this process, the bacteria are put through a giant "strainer." Although some bacterial chains are broken, which reduces activity, and the supernatant is separated, which reduces the effectiveness of the bacteria, ultrafiltration does not damage fragile cell walls and is generally easier on bacteria than centrifuging. However, although ultrafiltration may be less damaging to the bacteria, it is still an inferior processing method, resulting in an inferior product.

The biggest problem with both the centrifuging and ultrafiltration processes is that in both methods, the beneficial supernatant is stripped away. Without the supernatant, the antimicrobial byproducts and a host of other beneficial substances of the bacteria are lost. This means less extra benefits for you and a loss of protection for the bacteria themselves. Without their growing medium to act as a buffer, the bacteria is left naked and exposed to the killing power of stomach acids on their way through the digestive system. It also means that any friendly bacteria that arrive at their ultimate destination are stripped of microbe-fighting substances and the food source they need to live.

No matter how well they were growing before they were separated from the supernatant, any bacteria that survive the separation process and the onslaught of stomach acids in their travels, end up in your gastrointestinal tract weak, hungry, naked, and without a ready-made food source. Centrifuged or ultrafiltrated bacteria simply aren't equipped to take on the "bad guys" that continually assault your body.

Full-Culture Processing Method

The most desirable of the bacteria processing methods is the full-culture production method. Together, the entire bacterial mass, including its supernatant are freeze-dried and packaged. This type of processing results in a true quality product.

Freeze-Drying (Lyophilization)

The supernatant is indispensable to your friendly bacteria. How would you like to find yourself in a new country and discover that before you were able to eat you had to grow your own food? You'd be very weak before your garden was ready for harvest. Think of this analogy if someone tells you that the friendly bacteria can "grow" their own supernatant inside your body. There is no research to support what type of supernatant will be grown—the supernatant is only as good as its food source.

The best way to capture the living colonies of beneficial bacteria and sustain them for a predetermined length of time is through a freeze-drying process called lyophilizing. This lightning-fast biochemical process dries the bacteria by freezing it within a vacuum. All that is removed is the water.

Proprietary freeze-drying of the bacteria preserves the supernatant, which helps protect the friendly bacteria as well. The supernatant provides a natural buffer for the friendly bacteria that enables them to survive gastric acids. It also gives supplemental beneficial bacteria everything they need to succeed in setting up colonies, because they remain in their natural environment. Researchers have demonstrated that many of the beneficial properties of probiotic microorganisms can be attributed to the active enzymes and powerful antimicrobial substances the friendly bacteria have produced in the supernatant.

It is immeasurably more expensive to freeze-dry the bacteria and the supernatant together, but it is the only way to capture the living colonies of beneficial bacteria and sustain them for a predetermined length of time. Freeze-drying puts the bacteria into an arrested state of growth. When the bacteria reach their new home in your gastrointestinal tract, they are ready to take up residence immediately.

Remember, bacteria are microscopic and commonly represent only three percent of the finished bottled product in most commercial brands. Freeze-drying three percent bacteria concentrate that has been processed through centrifugation or ultrafiltration, then blending it in a cheap filler such as malto-dextrin (about 50 cents a pound) makes the finished product inexpensive to produce. It is economical for the consumer, as well, but don't forget that you get what you pay for—an inferior product.

The most desirable product is one that has been processed using the full-culture method. These bacteria cells along with their valuable supernatant are freeze-dried at a production cost of approximately $8.00 per pound. This may result in a more expensive product, but know that it is a high-quality one—not one that is made with 97 percent cheap fillers.

THE RIGHT BACTERIAL COUNT

How many bacteria do you need? As far as beneficial bacteria are concerned, "the more the merrier" definitely applies. Dr. J.L. Rasic, writing on both *L. acidophilus* and bifidobacteria, states, "An effective supplement should contain a minimum of *hundreds of millions* to *billions* of bacterial cells per day."

This may be easy to say, but difficult to really comprehend. It is hard to visualize 1 million, let alone 1 billion anything. To get an idea of the vast difference between the two, consider this: It would take the second hand of your clock about two weeks, just under fourteen days, to tick off 1 million seconds. But the same second hand would take almost half a lifetime, thirty-two years, before 1 billion seconds pass by.

To be effective, a probiotic supplement should contain a guaranteed count of at least 1 billion bacteria of a specific super strain of the right species. Remember, you can't substitute one bacteria for another. You need beneficial bacteria that can take up residence in both your small intestine (*L. acidophilus*) and large intestine (*B. bifidum*), as well as the friendly "traveling" bacteria (*L. bulgaricus*) that supports the other two, as well as offering special benefits of its own.

THE POTENCY GUARANTEE

If you are not in the habit of reading labels carefully, be sure to start when selecting probiotics. Very few probiotic products provide a guarantee of potency through a clearly-stated expiration date. Often, what you will find is a statement showing a bacteria count at the time

Avoid Probiotics
with FOS

Fructooligosaccharides, more commonly known as FOS, is a class of simple carbohydrates found naturally in certain plants, such as Jerusalem artichokes, onions, and bananas. Virtually, all of the FOS added to probiotic products in the United States is chemically manufactured. A Japanese process is utilized in turning white, bleached cane sugar, by the action of a fungal enzyme, into FOS—a sugar polymer that our bodies cannot digest.

FOS, known in Japan as Meioligo and in scientific terms as neosugar, is used as a sweetening agent, flavor enhancer, bulking agent, and humectant. As a low-calorie sucrose-replacement, FOS is used in cookies, cakes, breads, candies, dairy products, and some beverages. FOS is also added to some Japanese health foods to promote the growth of beneficial bacteria in the gastrointestinal tract

In 1990, Coors Biotech, in an effort to introduce FOS into the food chain of the United States, prepared a GRAS (generally recognized as safe) petition to include FOS as a human food ingredient. As several years of FOS-safe food sales are needed before this approval, the probiotic market was chosen as an easy, nonthreatening way to get the product "out there." The health food industry became an ideal test market.

The addition of FOS in probiotic products is becoming a common practice. Many probiotic manufacturers claim FOS is beneficial in that it feeds the friendly bacteria. Those who manufacture high-quality probiotics, however, do not believe in using FOS. Instead, their products require one important component—the valuable supernatant, which naturally and specifically provides food for the bacteria. (See The All-Important Supernatant on page 115.)

Prudent probiotic manufacturers are concerned with the safety issue of FOS. According to a study conducted by the Joint Expert Committee on Food Additives (JECFA) of the Food and Agricultural Organization and World Health Organization (FAO/WHO), the consumption of FOS may cause intestinal problems, such as bloating, abdominal pain, and copious amounts of gas.

> *There are a number of additional reasons why some manufacturers of high-quality probiotics do not add FOS to their products. They are:*
>
> - *FOS is manufactured by chemical synthesis. The ingredient is, therefore, not natural, but a chemical additive and may pose toxicological dangers.*
> - *FOS is a sugar derivative, therefore, those with a yeast infection should avoid it.*
> - *The stability of FOS is poor. The industrial production of purified FOS is a problem and still in the developmental stage.*
> - *FOS is inert in the mouth and small intestine because it is not digestible (similar to oelstra). It is digested in the colon by the bacteria and may, therefore, change the metabolic activity of the colon, resulting in abnormal functions.*
> - *FOS stimulates the growth of Klebsiella and possibly other pathogenic organisms. In one study, Klebsiella has been associated with the autoimmune disease ankylosing spondylitis.*
> - *FOS is known to be species as well as strain specific. In other words, not all beneficial bacteria like the FOS diet.*
>
> *As always, be an educated consumer when choosing probiotic products. Read labels. Choose only high-quality products that include the beneficial supernatant, and avoid those that include FOS.*

of manufacture. This statement, which is not good enough, is a clear indication that the seller cannot guarantee potency past the time the bacteria was packaged. Such a product may be useless by the time you take it.

Remember, too, that if the product was processed through centrifugation or ultrafiltration, not only has the supernatant been discarded, leaving the bacteria weak and unable to survive for very long, but the total number of bacteria shown on the label may be artificially inflated because broken bits and pieces of bacteria may be included in the total count. Dr. Khem Shahani warns, "Many products contain extremely low levels of living acidophilus cells, and those that are living are unstable. Many manufacturers give the number of living cells at the time the product was formulated, or the bottle filled. But

---

Probiotics for Pets

If you're a pet lover who recognizes that love isn't always enough, you'll be glad to know that there is a special line of probiotic supplements for cats, dogs, and horses. If this strikes you as odd, please think again. Many families give their own "people probiotics" to their pets with great success. If you want to give your animals the benefits of probiotics, please ask the staff at your health food store about probiotics for pets. The best of these products provide L. acidophilus NAS super strain, and are held to the same quality standards as the best "people products."

Because animals aren't always eager to take their medicine, probiotics for pets come in a gel that will cause your favorite pet to "lick his lips." Everyone has a story to tell about a beloved animal who could wolf down a bowl full of food and spit out a capsule of medication that has been buried in it. Believe me, animals can't spit out gel. Probiotics for pets comes with a dispenser marked in increments, along with clear instructions explaining how to determine the most effective amount to give your animals.

---

after manufacturing and storage, the count goes down, and the number of living cells can drop as low as zero."

Please take the time to read probiotic labels carefully. This is a good time to be skeptical. Insist on a product that gives you a potency guarantee in the billions and a printed potency expiration date. And be sure that "not centrifuged" and "contains supernatant" appear on the label.

THE RIGHT PACKAGING

Light, moisture, and heat destroy bacterial potency. Quality probiotics should be protected by heavy amber glass bottles that shield the living organisms from light and moisture, which is especially damaging. Even opaque plastic bottles that block light are not good enough. The amber glass bottles not only provide the optimum environment for product stability, but the heavy glass protects the product from moisture, which is able to seep through virtually all plastic bottles.

Most companies with probiotic products on the market use two-piece hard gelatin capsules or enteric-coated capsules. Some hard gel caps are high in moisture, which can damage the bacteria significantly. Enteric-coated capsules, which are coated with shellac, are designed to break apart in the stomach and release the beneficial bacteria into the intestinal tract. However, if the person's digestive system isn't working properly, the capsules may not break apart but remain intact, leaving the body in the same form in which they entered it. (Although enteric-coated capsules are effective carriers for a number of drugs, their efficacy in protecting bacteria has yet to be proven.)

Selected hard gelatin capsules are best, especially those that have been treated with a sophisticated modified-release system. These capsules take five to seven hours to break apart and are affected by the varying pH balances in the gastrointestinal tract as they travel. They begin breaking up and releasing bacteria in the stomach and continue the process in the small and large intestines until all of the beneficial bacteria has been released into the body.

REVOLUTIONARY PROBIOTIC PRODUCTS FOR THE TWENTY-FIRST CENTURY

I have said that by the year 2000 everyone will be as familiar with probiotic bacteria as they are with vitamins today. I firmly believe that what you are learning in this book constitutes what will be hailed as the breakthrough "medicine" of the twenty-first century.

With that in mind, here's a look at two true revolutionary breakthrough products in the field of probiotics that are available right now. Both involve new proprietary technology and are unique in the field. One product contains the "big-three" trinity of probiotics in one convenient capsule. The other is actually a trio of separate, selected bacterial super strains in both powder and capsule forms.

Big Three Trio—One Convenient Capsule

The convenience of having all three super strains of the most effective friendly bacteria in one capsule is a recent technological breakthrough. As copycat products may exist, be sure to seek out the probiotic product that provides 5 billion *L. acidophilus* (NAS super strain), 20 billion *B. bifidum* (Malyoth super strain), and 5 billion *L. bulgaricus* (LB-51 super strain) per capsule.

You must also be very careful to select a combination product that has been formulated with the proper delivery system. Without it, the bacteria compete with each other for nutrients and growing room. This competitive atmosphere results in mass destruction and a dramatically reduced count of live bacteria.

There is only one effective product that employs a specially blended oil-matrix system that keeps the bacteria separate and noncompetitive. This system allows the three super strains to happily coexist side-by-side in capsule form. It also protects the bacteria against the onslaught of gastric juices as they pass through the stomach. Tests show that organisms protected by the oil-matrix carrier survived one hour in a simulated gastric juice environment with no cell loss. Consisting of sunflower oil and vitamin E that has had all of the oxygen and water removed, this medium creates an ideal anaerobic (oxygen-free) environment.

After the bacteria are grown, it takes three days to remove all the water and oxygen from the oil matrix. Then it takes another three days to introduce each of the bacteria separately, one species at a time, into their new environment. Each tiny bacteria is literally "microenrobed" with the matrix. They exist in their own special "bubble," and never come in contact with one another. This process protects and totally separates the acidophilus, bifidum, and bulgaricus cells from each other until they are called into action in your intestinal tract.

In order for this probiotic combo to be effective, it must be produced in "clean rooms" maintained at the highest pharmaceutical standards under nitrogen-flush conditions that insure the absence of oxygen. In an oxygen-free atmosphere, the bacteria in their "bubbles" are placed in hard-shell gelatin capsules. The capsules themselves then must be double-sealed and given special protection that shields them completely from air and moisture. This extra pampering is necessary. Unfortunately, this final, critical stage must be performed in Europe, where the necessary special technology is available. Of course, this adds to the cost of the product, but it is the only way to make absolutely certain that the bacteria remain separate and viable until you take them.

If you see a probiotic combo on the shelf in your favorite health food store, be sure to read its label. While the product may look good, it could be weak and ineffective. Look for a product that contains *L. acidophilus*, *B. bifidum*, and *L. bulgaricus* in the amounts mentioned above. Be sure the bacteria are in a sunflower-oil matrix and encased in a two-piece hard gelatin capsule.

With a quality combination product, you can easily achieve quick results in establishing or facilitating optimal performance of your friendly flora. During the first two weeks, take one capsule three times daily just before meals. Thereafter, or for maintenance purposes, take one capsule daily for life.

Selected Probiotic Strains

The other revolutionary product is a trio of individual probiotic super strains in both powder and capsule forms. The trio includes *L. acidophilus* (DDS-1 or NAS super strain), *B. bifidum* (Malyoth super strain), and *L. bulgaricus* (LB-51 super strain). For optimum results, I always recommend including selected powders in your probiotic program as well as capsules. Powdered probiotics begin working immediately upon ingestion, while capsulized probiotics are designed to open in the intestinal tract.

Taking both capsules and powders is important in maintaining a healthy gastrointestinal tract, which insures your body the fullest protection. Remember, your gastrointestinal tract really starts at your mouth, which houses over 600 bacterial species.

Powdered probiotics are most effective in the mouth, esophagus, and upper small intestine. The oil-matrix capsule was designed to deliver large amounts of the beneficial bacteria to the lower small intestine and the large intestine.

The optimal probiotic supplementation for the maintenance of your friendly bacteria is ½ teaspoon of each super strain powder twice a day along with one oil-matrix "trinity" capsule.

SUMMING IT UP—DETERMINING A PRODUCT'S WORTH

In real estate, it's said that the three things that determine the worth of a property are location, location, and location. In probiotics, the three things that determine a product's worth are quality, quality, and quality.

The only way you can be sure of getting quality probiotic products is to know—and be able to trust—your supplier. Remember, you must have literally billions of bacteria that are alive and well before you can expect to receive any benefits. Make sure you select probiotics that

Probiotics
Powders or Capsules?

Probiotic supplements are available in a number of forms, the two most popular being capsules and freeze-dried powders. As a consumer, there are a few bits of information that can help you decide which form is best to suit your individual needs.

- *Freeze-dried powders.* All probiotic supplements come in *freeze-dried powders, which are generally taken in unchilled filtered water. When purchasing powders, be sure each product contains a single bacterial super strain. In powdered form, the friendly bacteria get into the gastrointestinal sytem faster than when taken in capsules. In addition to simple personal preference, this form is recommended for children and those who have difficulty swallowing capsules.*

  As the powders begin working immediately in the mouth, esophagus, and stomach, they are especially helpful for treating such problems as nausea, stomach upset, and acid reflux. Mixed in water, then slowly sipped through a straw, the friendly bacteria are able to get to the source of the problem quickly. Powders are also the most convenient form when preparing topical pastes for acne and diaper rash.

- *Capsules.* Certain strains of L. acidophilus and B. bifidum, *including the super strains, are sold individually in capsule form. (L. bulgaricus is not yet available in capsules.) Generally, capsules are preferred over powders because of their convenience.*

- *Wafers.* Convenient L. bulgaricus wafers are great to nibble on *at the first sign of nausea, indigestion, or acid reflux. They are also good for curbing appetites. Because of their convenient form, you can slip them easily into a purse or carry them in a briefcase when traveling away from home.*

- *Liquid.* As virtually all liquid probiotics lose their potency within *two weeks after they are produced, they should be avoided. (Most liquids don't even make it to store shelves within that period of time.) Liquid acidophilus, for example, must be handled like a perishable dairy product, with distinct expiration dates and strict refrigerated handling at all time. The reality is that liquid acidopilus products are generally handled like powdered supplements, with little or no refrigeration and a pull date that is often one year or longer after packaging. Some companies resort to adding bufferering agents to prevent the product from becoming sour or bitter. Such additives interfere with the bacteria's optimum performance.*

Overall, liquid probiotics are the most misrepresented products on the market. They provide little, if any, benefits to the consumer. More stringent standards must be maintained and adhered to by manufacturers.

retain the all-important supernatant growth medium, too. This growth base contains beneficial products that will greatly benefit both you and the friendly bacteria.

Search out standardized probiotic products. Most probiotic products that you find in stores are not standardized. Verified by independent laboratory analysis, a standardized probiotic product is one that has a DNA "fingerprint" taken of the primary culture. Production cultures must be taken from the same primary culture each time. To prove that no mutation of the organism has occurred, a DNA fingerprint must be taken of the production culture and matched to the finished product. Each bacteria must be grown in the same growth medium each time it is produced, and the label should assure you of that fact. Only probiotics that have been standardized and certified by laboratory analysis can give you predictable results every time.

Be sure you select products from a reputable source. Far too many of the probiotics in the marketplace are put out by private-label distributors who have purchased bacteria from growers who specialize in selling mass-produced cultures grown from inexpensive strains of bacteria. Commercially grown, mass-produced bacteria don't measure up to the home-grown, hand-raised super strains you want. Then, too, at least 80 percent of the probiotic products on the market carry labels that do not accurately reflect the contents of the product.

Learn to be a label reader. Some producers use questionable soil bacteria such as *B. laterosporum* (which cannot be substituted for a human strain) or *Enterococcus faecium* (formerly known as *Strepto-*

coccus faecium) in their cultures. While some strains of *E. faecium* may be helpful, others have been shown to cause food poisoning. In 1995, the National Nutritional Foods Association (NNFA) resolved to research *E. faecium* further before endorsing it for human use. Manufacturers, however, continue to use it in their supplemental lactobacillus mixtures, because it is considerably cheaper and easier to grow than other lactobacteria.

Steer clear of products containing *Lactobacillus sporagenes*, which is the former name for a soil bacteria known as *B. coagulous*. Soil bacteria supplements can be dangerous substitutes for real human probiotics. Under certain conditions, the bacteria can turn toxic. Some of these organisms, which also include *B. laterosporus*, are used to illicit some type of reaction when ingested, so consumers believe they are getting their money's worth. For example, certain soil bacteria supplements may cause candidiasis symptoms to subside. However, once the supplement is stopped, the symptoms return, often stronger than before.

Know that the best probiotic producers offer a complete line of quality probiotics. If you see a few lonely bottles of bargain-priced acidophilus on the shelf without a full array of other products of the same brand to keep them company, be suspicious. You may have stumbled onto an entrepreneur who slaps his or her private label on the least expensive "something-dophilus" available. In choosing probiotics, price is often an indication of quality. This is one case in which you get what you pay for.

Remember, if you expect to receive the documented benefits reported in this book, you must select the highest quality probiotics in the marketplace.

Part Two

The Disorders

As you have seen in Part One, many health problems are related, in some way or other, to a deficiency of the beneficial bacteria in your gastrointestinal tract. Unless the friendly bacteria are vigilant in carrying out their duties, all kinds of things can go wrong. For example, you would probably never guess that there is a connection between a deficiency of friendly bacteria and such diverse disorders as acne and skin conditions, anxiety and depression, dental cavities and gum disease, headaches (including migraines), radiation sickness, and stress; but there is.

Although every system of your body is vital to your health and well being, no single system is more important than your gastrointestinal tract. The state of the friendly bacteria in your intestines affects just about every part of your body, including your mental state. When your small and large intestines are fully colonized with friendly bacteria, your first line of defense is solidly in place; your body is ready to stand firm against harmful bacteria.

Part Two opens with some general guidelines on taking probiotics and is followed by an easy-to-read A-to-Z listing of common illnesses and conditions that can result from friendly bacteria deficiency. Each entry includes a brief description of the disorder, as well as its causes and symptoms. Recommended probiotic regimens are provided for each.

General Guidelines for Taking Probiotics

One of the best things about the right probiotic products is that it's impossible to take too many. Unlike drugs, herbs, and even some vitamins and minerals, there's no way to take a dangerous overdose of probiotics. Feel free to mix and match the "big three" trinity of friendly bacteria—*L. acidophilus*, *B. bifidum* and *L. bulgaricus*—in powders and/or capsules according to your needs. In quality probiotics, it's truly "the more the merrier."

If a particular health problem, including those discussed in this book, indicates a need for increased supplementation of probiotics, use the amounts suggested on the label as a starting point and increase your intake as needed. Friendly bacteria are not toxic substances. You may increase the amount you take and the frequency with which you take them for a lifetime.

When using probiotics in powdered form, it is very important to mix it with filtered water only, not tap water. Tap water is not only filled with a variety of contaminants, it's highly chlorinated. While chlorine is helpful in destroying dangerous bacteria, it kills beneficial bacteria as well. Filtered water is the best choice for drinking and cooking, too. If you are installing a water filtration system in your home or business, make sure the system takes out pesticides and chlorine but leaves the minerals. Using a filtration system is better than buying bottled water because many bottled waters do not include minerals. It is also important that you mix probiotic powders in water that is the correct temperature—unchilled. If the water is too cold, the bacterial will hibernate, and it won't activate quickly.

You must be very careful when selecting probiotic products. Quality must be your number-one priority. Positive results are achieved only if probiotics are cultured with the right species and super strains of friendly bacteria. (For detailed information on choosing the best-quality products, see Chapter 10.)

Read labels! When choosing probiotic supplements, always choose the highest quality possible. Keep the following guidelines in mind when making your selection:

- When choosing capsules, be sure that each one contains a guaranteed count of at least 2 billion bacteria of the best specific strain. Powdered products should contain at least 2 billion bacteria per ½ teaspoon amount.

- If you are choosing a product that contains all three super strains in one capsule, be sure to select one that has been formulated with an oil-matrix carrier, which effectively keeps the bacteria separate and noncompetitive. The highest quality products offer 5 billion *L. acidophilus* (DDS-1 or NAS super strain), 20 billion *B. bifidum* (Malyoth super strain), and 5 billion *L. bulgaricus* (LB-51 super strain) per capsule.

- Be wary of combination powdered products that claim to have a wide variety of different bacterial species without giving a specific bacterial count. The product may contain very little of the bacteria you want. It is best to choose powdered products that contain only one strain.

- Be sure the product includes the bacteria's growth medium—the supernatant (see The All-Important Supernatant on page 115).

- Check the product label for a guaranteed expiration date. Beware of any label that states a potency guarantee "at the time of manufacture" or "shipment." Such guarantees are unrelated to the bacterial potency at the time you buy the product. They mislead and confuse the consumer.

- Choose only products that have the words "not centrifuged" on the label. (For further information on the centrifugation process, see page 122.)

Keeping these points in mind will enable you to make educated choices in your search for high-quality products.

Probiotic Use During Antibiotic Treatment

Although antibiotics are capable of killing harmful bacteria, unfortunately, they kill friendly bacteria as well. And when friendly bacteria are weak or in small numbers, the field is left wide open for such microbes as Candida albicans—a yeast that, when given the opportunity, proliferates and transforms into a dangerous fungus that can wreak havoc with the immune system (see Candidiasis entry in Part Two).

Another growing problem with antibiotics is that a number of harmful bacteria, such as certain strains of the insidious Staphylococcus aureus, (see inset on page 208) are becoming resistent to them. For example, Vancomycin—the biggest gun in the antibiotic arsenal—is unable to treat a number of once-treatable bacterial infections.

There are times, however, when you may need antibiotics. It is during this time, more than ever, that taking supplements of the "bigthree" probiotic super strains (L. acidophilus, B. bifidum, and L. bulgaricus) are important. Although antibiotics and probiotics should be taken concurrently, they are not to be taken at the exact same time. In order for the probiotics to be most effective, take them at least two hours after each dose of antibiotics. Once the antibiotic treatment is over, be sure to double or triple the probiotic regimen for ten days to two weeks. This will help your gastrointestinal tract reestablish its friendly flora.

When taking antibiotics, the following probiotic regimen is recommended:

- *Two hours following each prescribed dose of antibiotics, take 2 capsules each of L. acidophilus, and B. bifidum (or 1 to 2 teaspoons powder), along with 1 teaspoon L. bulgaricus powder mixed in 6 to 8 ounces unchilled filtered water. For added strength, also take 1 combination capsule that contains all three super strains in an oil matrix carrier, three times daily.*
- *Before bed, take another dose of the powders as described above.*
- *If experiencing stomach upset, mix another dose as described above and sip it slowly*
- *For at least two weeks following antibiotic treatment, double or triple the above regimen.*

Acne. *See also* Skin Problems.

Although many adults are victims of acne, it is primarily an affliction of the teen years. Affecting 30 percent of teenage females and 44 percent of the males, acne is the most common skin disease of adolescence. One out of every five patients who consults a dermatologist has acne. In most of these cases, a chronic skin infection also exists.

Although there are as many as eleven different forms of acne, the condition is basically a dysfunction of the sebaceous (oil-producing) glands of the skin—often the result of bacterial contamination, hormone imbalance, nutritional deficiencies, emotional stress, or poor hygiene. Any combination of these factors can give rise to the condition. Common medical treatments for various forms of acne include vitamin-A therapy, antibiotics, benzyl benzoate, topical cleansing, chemical peels, and dermabrasion. All of these treatments are effective to a degree, but putting the friendly bacteria to work on the problem provides additional help.

In 1964, Dr. R.H. Siver reported on his work in a paper entitled, "Lactobacillus for the Control of Acne," which was published in the Journal of the Medical Society of New Jersey. Dr. Siver states, "Lactobacilli are a safe, simple, 80 percent effective treatment for acne, especially in boys and girls under the age of 18."

Dr. Siver documented an improvement in patients suffering from acne who were taking lactobacteria for a gastrointestinal condition. The eight-day course of treatment included two or three tablets of *L. acidophilus* and *L. bulgaricus* daily, taken with milk, followed by two weeks without supplementation. When necessary, the course of treatment was repeated again. In most cases, improvement was seen within the first two weeks.

Dr. Siver was not surprised to find that acidophilus and bulgaricus quickly cleared up the intestinal afflictions troubling his patients, but the fact that the skin conditions cleared up as well was unexpected. No doubt this effect can be attributed to the general cleansing action of the friendly bacteria.

Dr. Siver reported an 80 percent success rate in treating over 300 cases of patients with acne. Of the patients ranging in age from 18 to 25, half had what he termed "reasonable success." The other half, all under age 18, had what Dr. Siver called "excellent results."

Russian and Bulgarian doctors have successfully used topical acidophilus or bulgaricus pastes to treat acne for decades. You can make a similar paste—start by mixing 1 level teaspoon of *L. bulgaricus* powder with enough fresh aloe vera (scraped from the inside of a leaf) and distilled water to form a smooth, spreadable paste. After washing your face, gently pat it dry with a clean towel. Apply the probiotic paste to the entire face and neck area. Leave the paste on for twenty minutes or longer before rinsing it off gently with a clean washcloth and warm water. In addition to clearing up acne, this paste speeds gentle facial exfoliation, while smoothing and softening the skin's texture. It also tightens pores and softens lines and wrinkles.

RECOMMENDED PROBIOTIC REGIMEN

- Take 1 capsule each of *L. acidophilus* and *B. bifidum* (or ½ teaspoon each powder), along with ½ teaspoon *L. bulgaricus* powder mixed in 6 to 8 ounces unchilled filtered water, two times daily. May be increased to 2 capsules *L. acidophilus* and *B. bifidum*, and 1 teaspoon *L. bulgaricus*, three times daily.

- Instead of the above regimen, take 1 or 2 combination capsules that contain all three super strains in an oil-matrix carrier, once a day.

- Apply topical homemade probiotic paste (described in entry), once a day for at least two weeks, depending on the severity of the acne.

- For maintenance, continue taking the above oral regimen two times daily, and continue using the probiotic paste twice a week. Also apply probiotic face cream (page 202) daily in the morning and evening.

NOTE: For choosing the highest quality probiotics, see guidelines beginning on page 137.

Aging Skin.

See Skin Problems.

Ankylosing Spondylitis.

Ankylosing spondylitis (AS), sometimes called "poker spine" or "bamboo spine," is a long-term rheumatic disorder that affects the joints of the spine and is characterized by pain and inflammation. Hundreds of thousands of Americans are affected with AS, with millions of others suffering from related symptoms. Often, early sufferers of AS self-diagnose their symptoms as nothing more than nagging back pain or early arthritis.

The first symptoms of ankylosing spondylitis usually begin with inflamed joints of the spine that eventually stiffen, then progress to an ankylosis (joining together) of the vertebrae. The damage is caused by a gradual encroachment of each vertebrae to the ones above and below it. The spine may become fused into a bent position, often to such a degree that the individual cannot look forward without extreme difficulty. The bones of the pelvis may also join together, resulting in pain and great difficulty in sitting. If the joints between the spine and ribs are affected, the chest wall's ability to expand will be limited and may cause breathing difficulty and heart problems.

Medical treatment for AS includes drugs to relieve pain, physical therapy to keep the spine as erect as possible, and, in advanced cases, surgery to straighten a spine that has become badly bent.

Human tissues are scientifically typed according to their biochemical and cellular characteristics. One tissue type, designated B27, is present in almost 100 percent of people suffering from ankylosing spondylitis. The research of Dr. Alan Ebringer of King's College Hospital in London, shows why this is important.

Dr. Ebringer theorized that the body's immune system could make a mistake in its efforts to get rid of an undesirable bacteria and be fooled into attacking its own tissues instead. To confirm his theory, Dr. Erbinger and his research team typed different bacteria taken from the intestinal tract of AS patients in order to identify the one bacteria that most closely matched B27 tissue type characteristics. The bacterial culprit was *Klebsiella*. The researchers showed that the immune system could easily mistake B27 tissue cells for *Klebsiella*. Once the similarity between *Klebsiella* and B27 tissues was established, the researchers next examined the feces of AS patients to test their theory.

They discovered that in the active stages of the disease, when inflammation was at its highest peak, *Klebsiella* levels in the stool, and antibody levels of *Klebsiella* in the blood, were much higher than in the periods when the disease was relatively calm. Those antibodies, designed to rid the body of *Klebsiella*, also attacked B27 tissue cells. In other words, as the immune system mounted an attack to rid the body of the *Klebsiella* bacteria, it became confused and attacked the body's own B27 cells instead.

The correct type of probiotic strains can play an important preventive role in AS. By successfully competing with *Klebsiella* for attachment sites on the intestinal wall, *L. acidophilus*, *B. bifidum*, and *L. bulgaricus* can prevent or curb an overgrowth of this harmful bacteria. Daily supplementation with the recommended levels of probiotic super strains and a proper diet will produce positive results.

Klebsiella loves starch and sugar, including FOS (see inset on page 126); therefore, it is important to eliminate bread, pasta, cereals, rice, and potatoes, as well as all sugary foods from your diet. You should consume vegetables, fruits, eggs, cheese, fish, and meat in amounts necessary to maintain your ideal weight.

RECOMMENDED PROBIOTIC REGIMEN

- Take 1 capsule each of *L. acidophilus* and *B. bifidum* (or ½ teaspoon each powder), along with ½ teaspoon *L. bulgaricus* powder mixed in 6 to 8 ounces unchilled filtered water, three times daily. Take 10 to 30 minutes before meals.

- Instead of the above regimen, take 1 or 2 combination capsules that contain all three super strains in an oil-matrix carrier, once a day.

NOTE: For choosing the highest quality probiotics, see guidelines beginning on page 137.

Anxiety. *See also* Depression; Stress.

Everyone experiences anxiety—an unpleasant emotional state that is a direct response to stress. Closely associated with fear, anxiety can come on suddenly or gradually over a period of time. Lasting from a few seconds to years, anxiety can range in intensity from "butterflies in the stomach" to a full-blown panic attack complete with shortness of breath, increased heartbeat, sweating, and dizziness.

A certain level of anxiety is normal, actually important, as it appropriately cautions us to dangerous situations around us. Most people are able to handle anxiety, keeping it within a normal realm. Some people, however, are overwhelmed with the fear and panic that arises from anxiety. When anxiety occurs at inappropriate times, or lasts so long that it interferes with a person's normal activities, it is considered a disorder.

Common symptoms of anxiety disorder may include restlessness, irritability, muscle tension, and insomnia. Worry generated by a person with an anxiety disorder is often general in nature and difficult to control. Common worries, which are taken to an inappropriately intense level, often involve health, money, and work.

Sudden anxiety, fear, or stress results in the release of adrenaline, which puts the body on alert—ready for "fight or flight." Quickened heartbeat, dilated pupils, and shortness of breath are physical changes that occur almost instantaneously and intensely. Additionally, the blood rushes from the digestive system to the muscles, where it may be needed in response to the need to possibly "fight." A continued pattern of this adrenaline rush can result in damaging effects to the digestive system, especially the large intestine and colon.

Both anxiety and stress can be controlled through behavioral therapy, breathing techniques, meditation, and visualization. In addition, it's important to keep your friendly bacteria, especially lactobacilli, strong. In sufficient numbers, lactobacilli can help encourage a relaxed state. You see, during fermentation, lactobacilli release tryptophan, which produces the calming neurotransmitter seratonin. Tryptophan is found in milk, which is why drinking a glass of warm milk is a traditional cure for insomnia. The tryptophan in the milk has a relaxing, calming effect. True yogurt and other cultured milk products contain even higher levels of tryptophan, and high quality lactobacteria supplements contain the most.

While friendly lactobacteria may not directly alleviate anxiety and stress, its release of tryptophan (and resulting seratonin), may help to encourage a relaxed state. Taking high-quality supplemental lactobacilli can certainly be a positive step in dealing with anxiety.

RECOMMENDED PROBIOTIC REGIMEN

- Take 1 capsule each of L. *acidophilus* and B. *bifidum* (or ½ teaspoon powder), along with ½ teaspoon of L. *bulgaricus* powder mixed in 6 to 8 ounces unchilled filtered water, two times daily. May be increased to 2 capsules L. *acidophilus* and B. *bifidum* (or 1 teaspoon powder), along with 1 teaspoon L. *bulgaricus*, three times daily.
- Instead of the above regimen, take 1 or 2 capsules that contain all three super strains in an oil-matrix carrier, once a day.

NOTE: For choosing the highest quality probiotics, see guidelines beginning on page 137.

Botulism.

See Food Poisoning.

Bowel Toxicity.

See Toxic Bowel.

Cancer.

See Chapter 9; Radiation Poisoning.

Candidiasis.

Candidiasis is an infection caused by an overgrowth of the *Candida albicans* organism—a tiny, common yeast/fungus that lives in the mouth, throat, digestive tract, genitourinary tract, and on the skin of healthy persons. Under normal conditions, candida lives in healthy balance with the other bacteria in the body. It is essentially harmless, and in its yeast form is of no concern to us.

One of the most important responsibilities of your essential friendly bacteria is to keep *Candida albicans* under control. Active colonies of friendly bacteria are so vigilant in keeping these organisms from finding attachment sites, they seldom cause problems. Trouble begins, however, when the candida is allowed to rocket out of control and transform itself from an innocuous yeast into a dangerous pervasive fungus. Candida microbes are considered opportunistic—they jump at any opportunity to increase their territory.

Before going any further, it's important to understand the difference between yeast and fungi. Fungi are members of the plant kingdom. Yeasts as well as molds are a subgroup of the fungi family. These types of organisms live on the surfaces of living things, including fruits, vegetables, grains, and your skin. Unlike most plants, yeast has no roots and absorbs its nutrients from enzymes secreted by the organic material on which it lives. In small amounts, yeast is not harmful.

The candida yeast is an especially sneaky one. It can change from its rootless yeast form into an aggressive and tenacious fungus that puts down roots. The prongs (hyphea) of these roots can actually penetrate the lining of the intestines. When your intestinal walls are breached, partially digested food particles, toxic waste, yeast breakdown products, and other materials are able to pass directly into your bloodstream. Needless to say, these substances do not belong in your blood, so your immune system is called into action to fight these invaders. When this happens over and over, it causes a constant drain on your immune system cells, resulting in a general weakening of the immune system. In addition, eventually the immune system will be unable to handle the undigested food particles and your body will become allergic to that food.

The Herxheimer Reaction

True probiotic supplements as outlined in this book are not drugs and can be taken safely in larger amounts and greater frequencies than recommended. It is important to note, however, that if an individual is toxic—as in the case with candidiasis and toxic bowel sufferers, for instance—taking probiotics may elicit a "healing crisis" phenomenon. Also known as the Herxheimer reaction, this phenomenon is named after the German dermatologist Karl Herxheimer, M.D., who, together with another German dermatologist, Adolf Jarish, M.D., identified it.

You see, taking beneficial bacteria or an anti-fungal agent will cause an inhibition or die-off of harmful bacteria or fungi, which must exit the body via the feces or urine. When toxins are in large numbers, these exit routes are overcrowded and may be unable to accommodate the mass exit immediately. It is during this time that the individual may experience the Herxheimer Reaction—temporary toxic or allergic symptoms such as bloating, gas, and headaches.

Depending on the individual's toxicity level, it may be prudent to begin taking the minimum recommended probiotics, gradually increasing their amount and frequency. This will minimize any uncomfortable, although temporary, reactions. It is important to realize that these reactions are positive signs that the body is ridding itself of harmful organisms and their toxic byproducts.

MAJOR CAUSES

How is candida able to progress from its yeast form into a pathogenic fungus? There are many causes, a number of which are under your personal control. The major cause is the use of antibiotics. While effective in killing harmful bacteria, antibiotics destroy necessary friendly bacteria as well. (Candida organisms are unaffected by antibiotics.) Without friendly bacteria, your first line of defense against candida is eliminated, and these organisms are free to proliferate.

Because candida thrives in a sugar-laden environment, a high-sugar diet is another major cause for an infestation of this organism. Immunosuppressive drugs, such as steroids and birth control pills, and continuous infections, like Epstein-Barr virus and cytomegalovirus (a form of herpes), slow down immune system cells, making them less able to deal with candida overgrowth. Other causes for yeast overgrowth include hormonal changes associated with the menstrual cycle, pregnancy, and diabetes. Wearing nylon underwear is another common culprit. Synthetic materials cause increased perspiration, creating a warm, moist environment that is perfect for candida growth.

SYMPTOMS

What makes candidiasis so difficult to diagnose (and treat) is twofold. First, the illness itself can affect many different areas of the body, and, second, its wide variety of symptoms are characteristic of other illnesses and disorders. The following is but a partial list of the many symptoms and results of candidiasis:

- Candida overgrowth in the pockets of the stomach lining and intestinal tract commonly cause constipation and/or diarrhea, abdominal pain, gas, and bloating.
- In the mouth, candida overgrowth can cause thrush, a condition characterized by burning and/or spotted tongue, soreness in the corners of the mouth, canker sores, and bad breath.
- On the skin, candida overgrowth may result in athlete's foot, hives, jock itch, and fungal infections of the nails. Acne, psoriasis, and other chronic skin rashes are also common.
- An overgrowth of candida in the respiratory system may cause swollen membranes of the nose and throat, nagging cough, sore throat, congestion, clogged sinuses, and the development or increase of allergic reactions to things you eat, breathe, and/or touch.
- In the urinary tract, candida overgrowth may result in kidney and bladder infections.
- The reproductive systems of men, although not common trouble sites for yeast infections, can also be affected. Possible results are impaired sex drive, penile infections, and prostatitis.
- In the reproductive system of women, the increase in yeast can cause hormonal imbalances, premenstrual syndrome (PMS), menstrual irregularities, possible infertility, loss of sexual desire, abdominal pain, and vaginitis.

- The integration of candida toxins into hormonal secretions can affect the brain and nervous system. Symptoms may include fatigue, apathy, loss of energy, headaches, irritability, depression, anxiety, mood swings, and memory lapses.

- When the system is affected, likely symptoms can include unexplained weakness, aching, and/or swelling in muscles and joints; and possible numbness, burning, and/or tingling feeling in fingers and toes.

- Babies and children can also be targets of candida overgrowth, which commonly results in diaper rash. (For more information on babies and candidiasis, see Chapter 5.)

A rare form of the infection—chronic mucocutaneous candidiasis (CMC)—is linked to an inherited defect of the immune system. Usually occurring early in life (although it can develop as late as in the twenties), CMC causes skin sores, viral infections, and repeated lung involvement. Other problems associated with this unusual form of candidiasis include diabetes, Addison's disease, thyroid deficiency, and pernicious anemia. Some patients develop disfigurements and hormone imbalances as well. A hormone disorder of this type results in low levels of calcium, abnormal liver function, high blood sugar, iron deficiency, and abnormal vitamin B_{12} absorption.

DIAGNOSING CANDIDIASIS

There are two main laboratory methods for testing candidiasis—in one method, the candida antibodies are measured in the blood; in the other method, these organisms are examined in the stool. Unfortunately, neither test is very effective in making a diagnosis. This is because candida lives within all of us, so most of us also carry their antibodies. Identification of candida antibodies indicates only that the immune system has identified and defended us against the yeast at some time in our lives. And, when the immunoresponse is weak, which commonly occurs in someone taking immunosuppressive drugs or in those with a chronic immune system deficiency, testing the blood for candida antibodies may show little or no antibodies present, even though candida may be on a rampage.

Through his research and experiences, Dr. C. Orion Truss, the grandfather of candidiasis research and author of *Missing Diagnosis*, believes that laboratory testing is not the best route for identifying candidiasis. Knowing the major causes of candidiasis (see below) as well as its common symptoms (page 149) will be your best indicators. If you suspect you may be suffering from candida overgrowth, consult your health care provider and apprise him or her of your symptoms. After a review of your medical history (see Diagnosing Candidiasis: What Your Doctor Needs to Know, beginning on page 152), an evaluation can be made, and an anti-candida regimen can begin.

ARE YOU A CANDIDATE FOR CANDIDIASIS?

Identifying the factors that lead to an overgrowth of candida has proven to be a more reliable method of determining candida overgrowth than any of the standard tests. If you answer "yes" to any of the following questions, it is possible that you are in the throes of a candida assault, even if you are not currently suffering symptoms.

☐ Have you ever taken a course of broad-spectrum antibiotics for eight weeks or longer? Or more than three shorter courses of antibiotics within a year?

☐ Have you ever taken antibiotic treatment for acne for a month or longer?

☐ Have you ever taken steroids (cortisone, prednisone, or ACTH)?

☐ Have you used birth control pills for a year or more?

☐ Have you had more than one pregnancy?

☐ Do you eat a high-sugar diet?

☐ Have you ever been treated with immunosuppressive drugs?

☐ Have you ever had a chronic multiple infection (viral, bacterial, or parasitic), such as one that may occur in those with a chronically depressed immune system, including AIDS or ARC (AIDS-related complex)?

Positive answers to any of these questions, coupled with a display of some of the common symptoms of candidiasis (page 149), may indicate a candida overgrowth.

Diagnosing Candidiasis
What Your Doctor Needs to Know

In this age of specialization, the "family doctor" is an endangered species. At one time, not that long ago, most families went to one doctor who treated each family member as a patient, as well as a friend. This doctor knew the complete medical history of every member of the family. Today, the typical family sees many doctors, from internists to gynecologists, and urologists to pediatricians. Each one of these doctors concentrates on his or her own specialty. In other words, chances are that no one doctor has your complete medical history on file.

When you sit down with your favorite internist or general practitioner, be prepared to answer the following questions, which may help your doctor in determining if you are likely to have candidiasis:

☐ *Do you experience multiple allergic symptoms?*
☐ *Do you have an extreme sensitivity to chemical fumes, perfumes, or tobacco smoke?*
☐ *Do you seem to feel worse than usual (nauseous, achy, bloated, headachy, spaced out, irritable) after consuming yeasty or sugary foods or drinks?*
☐ *Do you crave sweet foods and/or alcohol?*
☐ *Do you have or did you ever have chronic acne?*
☐ *Do you suffer with frequent bouts of abdominal bloating, stomach distention, diarrhea, constipation, and/or anal itch?*
☐ *Are you generally tired and lethargic?*
☐ *Do you have a poor memory?*
☐ *Do you find it difficult to concentrate on the task at hand?*
☐ *Are you depressed?*
☐ *Do you have frequent upper respiratory tract infections, such as colds, postnasal drip, nagging coughs?*
☐ *Do you have athlete's foot, or a nail or skin fungus?*
☐ *Have you had an oral or vaginal yeast infection more than once?*
☐ *Do you frequently experience PMS (premenstrual syndrome) accompanied by fluid retention, irritability, mood swings, and so on?*
☐ *Do you generally suffer from menstrual cramps or pain?*

☐ *Do you have vaginal discharge, itching, and local irritation? Have you ever had vaginitis?*
☐ *Do you have recurrent or persistent cystitis, prostatitis, or endometriosis?*
☐ *Are you experiencing impotence or loss of sexual desire?*
☐ *Do you have muscle aches for no obvious reason?*
☐ *Are you experiencing tingling or numbness in your fingers and/or toes?*
☐ *Do you have swollen or aching joints for no obvious reason?*
☐ *Do you have erratic vision and/or spots before your eyes?*

Do not hesitate to discuss with your doctor any concerns you may have about a possible candida infection. It will help him or her in validating your suspicions.

TREATING CANDIDA OVERGROWTH

When treating candidiasis, it is important to watch your diet and avoid certain products. It is also advisable to take proper dietary supplements.

Watch the Foods You Eat and the Products You Use

Certain foods and a variety of products, including antibiotics, immunosuppressive drugs, steroids, and cigarettes, should be avoided if you have an overgrowth of candida.

If you have ever made bread, you know that yeast feeds on sugar. Because *Candida albicans* is a yeast, it thrives on sugar. To slow down the spread of candida, eliminate all refined and concentrated forms of sugar from your diet. Be aware that the natural sugars in fruits and fruit juices also feed the candida organism. Except for live yogurt and other foods based on lactobacillus fermentation (kefir, kumiss, etc.), yeasty and fermented foods, as well as foods that are likely to carry molds (nuts, some cheeses, and dried fruits), should be avoided.

The following is a listing of foods and a number of products that one should avoid when treating candidiasis. Be sure to check product labels carefully for "hidden" sugars.

- All sugar, including white sugar, brown sugar, honey, molasses, FOS (page 126), fructose, rice syrup, and corn syrup.
- Foods that include sugar, such as chocolate, candies, preserved fruits, jellies, jams, pickles, sauces, condiments, mayonnaise, breakfast cereals, ice cream, processed foods, and many prepared foods.
- Sugary drinks.
- Alcoholic beverages of any kind. Champagne and cordials have an unusually high sugar content.
- Fresh fruits and fruit juice. Even the natural sugar in fruit is a favorite food source of candida. The sugar in fruit juice is absorbed quickly by the body; if you must have your morning juice, dilute it with an equal amount of water and sip it slowly.
- Stimulants, including tea, coffee, cola, and cigarettes, which trigger the release of sugars in the body.
- All refined white flour products, including breads, prepared foods with a bread-crumb coating, buns, cakes, pastries, crackers, biscuits, noodles, and pastas. Choose whole grain varieties of these products instead. If you must have bread, select nonyeasted varieties.
- Foods containing citric acid (usually derived from yeast), including most canned or frozen citrus drinks.
- Multivitamin/multimineral supplements, unless from a guaranteed yeast-free source. Again, read labels carefully.
- Fermented foods, including soy sauce, cider, ginger ale, beer, wine, vinegar, sauerkraut, pickles, and relishes.
- Foods and products containing MSG (monosodium glutamate). Chinese foods as well as a number of processed foods often include MSG.
- Foods likely to carry hidden molds, including nuts, seeds, cheeses, and some Indian and Chinese teas.
- Meats or fish that have been cured, smoked, preserved, pickled, or processed in any way, including frankfurters, luncheon meats, and bacon.
- Antibiotics. Antibiotics kill the friendly bacteria that keep candida as well as other unwanted bacteria under control. Unless absolutely necessary, avoid antibiotics while you are trying to vanquish candida.
- Meats and poultry that come from animals raised on antibiotics. To

be sure you're not ingesting an unwanted dose of antibiotics along with your steak, choose organically raised meats and poultry.

- Nyastatin. This common antifungal medical drug is yeast-based. Research conducted at the Washington University School of Medicine shows that when nystatin treatment ends, a resurgence of yeast colonies often occurs, with more active colonies showing up than before treatment started.

It is important to avoid these foods and substances while you are fighting an active candida overgrowth. After three to four weeks, you can slowly begin reintroducing some of these foods back into your diet. Consider doing so on a rotating basis.

The rotation diet plan was designed to help anyone with symptoms of a food sensitivity or allergy, both of which are very common in those fighting candidiasis. This involves eating problem food families (all grains or all dairy products, for example), just once every four days or so. In this way, any adverse reaction to them is likely to lessen or disappear altogether. This also reduces the constant drain on your immune system that repeated allergic responses cause.

Take Proper Dietary Supplements

When caught in the throes of a candida rampage, you are faced with a two-fold task. First, you must give your body optimum nutrition, and, second, you must get the candida back to a manageable level.

Those suffering from candida overgrowth commonly have inadequate digestive function. There is every possibility that your protein requirements are not being met. For this reason, I suggest taking between five and fifteen grams of essential free-form amino acids with a glass of water at least thirty minutes before or ninety minutes after meals. To help insure smooth digestion of proteins, add a proteolytic (protein-digesting) enzyme to your supplement program— bromelain (from pineapple) and papain (from papaya) are two of the best, and both are health food store staples.

There are other dietary supplements that are helpful in the treatment of candida overgrowth. These include:

- *Biotin.* This important B-complex vitamin is produced by your beneficial bacteria. Remember, when candida has rocketed out of con-

trol, you know your friendly bacteria aren't fulfilling their obliga-
tions, including producing B-complex vitamins. Taking 500 mcg
daily with food is recommended until you are experiencing optimal health.

- *Caprylic (hexanoic) acid.* This coconut derivative is a champion antifungal. Unlike the yeast-derived antifungal drug nystatin, which
  actually encourages the quick growth of additional candida
  colonies once treatment has ended, caprylic acid has a totally
  benign effect. Several brands of caprylic acid are available. Read
  labels for recommended amounts.
- *Grapefruit seed extract.* This is an acceptable alternative to caprylic
  acid.
- *Garlic.* An ancient herbal medicinal, garlic is a well-known fungus
  fighter. Unless you're eating a lot of raw garlic, garlic supplements
  (many of which are odor-free) are recommended. Take 1 to 2 capsules three times daily with meals.
- *Olive oil.* This oil contains linoleic acid, an active antifungal. Driz-
  zle it on your salad, or try it on a chunk of whole-grain, nonyeasted bread. Take 1 tablespoon daily.
- *Germanium.* This nutrient has powerful antifungal properties. In
  addition, it enhances oxygenation, which increases energy. Recommended amount is 100 to 300 milligrams daily.
- *Aloe vera juice.* Another excellent antifungal. Several teaspoons in
  water daily is recommended.

If you experience gastrointestinal distress after eating and suffer
heartburn or abdominal discomfort, your stomach may not be secret-
ing enough hydrochloric acid to accomplish digestion. The answer is
not an acid reducer. You need to supplement your digestive acids to
bring them up to normal levels, not neutralize them. You can easily
supplement the production of digestive acid with betaine hydrochlo-
ride tablets or capsules from your health food store, or take a tablespoon of apple cider vinegar before eating.

L. bulgaricus is considered a powerful detoxifier. Take 1 heaping
teaspoon of *L. bulgaricus* powder (milk-based) in 8 ounces unchilled
filtered water before meals to aid protein and carbohydrate digestion.
If, however, your system is very toxic, this amount of *L. bulgaricus* will
cause a rapid die-off of harmful bacteria, which may result in a phys-

ical reaction, such as headache, gas, and bloating (see Herxheimer Reaction on page 148). Many individuals may opt for a milder dosage of *L. bulgaricus* and start out with ⅛ teaspoon of the powder, gradually increasing the amount over time.

To bring candida back to manageable levels, nothing is more important than probiotics. Research has shown that *L. acidophilus* produces substances that slow the growth of candida. When specific strains of acidophilus are added to petri dishes containing cultures of candida, they have demonstrated the ability to inhibit and stop the candida's growth.

In 1984, Japanese researchers tested the effects of bifidobacteria on twenty-seven leukemia patients who were receiving chemotherapy. Fecal analysis of these patients showed extremely high levels of candida—an average of 100 million organisms per gram of weight. After treatment with bifidobacteria, candida levels fell dramatically. In the sixteen patients given supplementary bifidobacteria, further analysis showed the presence of only about 10,000 candida organisms. The remaining eleven patients, who served as the control group, received no probiotic supplements and showed no change at all in their candida levels.

In his book, *Yeast Nutrition — Candida Albicans: An Unsuspected Problem*, Jeffrey Bland, professor of nutritional biochemistry at the University of Puget Sound in Tacoma, Washington, writes, "We have been very excited about an alternative therapy for the management of candida infection that avoids the use of anti-yeast medication. It is well-recognized that a disturbed flora of the gastrointestinal tract can establish a proper environment for yeast proliferation. By reinoculating the bowel with the proper symbiotic acid-producing bacteria, there is a reduction in the compatibility of the intestinal environment for the yeast proliferation. We have recently used an oral supplement of *Lactobacillus acidophilus* . . . this has been extremely successful in reducing *Candida albicans* in the intestinal tract."

RECOMMENDED PROBIOTIC REGIMEN

When beginning a probiotic regimen to combat candidiasis, it is important to realize that, depending on the level of toxicity, the die-off of toxins may result in the Herxheimer Reaction—gas, bloating, and possible headaches (see inset on page 148). Depending on the discomfort level you are willing to handle, it may be best to start with minimal amounts of probiotics, gradually increasing their amount and frequency as you see fit.

- Start with ½ teaspoon each of *L. acidophilus* and *B. bifidum* powders mixed together in 6 to 8 ounces unchilled filtered water (or 1 capsule of each), taken three times daily before meals.
- Take ¼ teaspoon *L. bulgaricus* powder mixed in 6 to 8 ounces unchilled filtered water, three times daily after meals.
- In addition to the above regimen, for increased strength, take 1 combination capsule that contains all three super strains in an oil-matrix carrier, once a day.
- Eat true yogurt that contains live cultures of both *L. bulgaricus* and *S. thermophilus* (if dairy products do not produce allergic reactions).

NOTE: For choosing the highest quality probiotics, see guidelines beginning on page 137.

Canker Sores. *See also* Cold Sores; Dental Problems.

Canker sores (apthous ulcers) are small, painful mouth sores. Unlike cold sores (fever blisters), which are caused by the contagious herpes simplex virus and usually appear on the hard part of the gums and outer part of the lips, canker sores are often found on the tongue, the soft part of the gums, and the inner cheeks and lips. Appearing suddenly, a canker sore begins as a red, ulcerated spot with a yellowish border. They can be as small as a pinhead or as large as a quarter, and they usually last anywhere from four to twenty days.

Occurring most often in females, canker sores can be caused by a number of factors, including poor oral hygiene, food allergies, nutritional deficiencies, viral infection, stress, and fatigue. Occasionally, canker sores are associated with Crohn's disease and candidiasis.

Under ideal circumstances, the natural flora of the mouth—including the right strains of the friendly bacteria—provide a barrier to canker sores. To help protect the normal alkaline environment of your mouth, practice good oral hygiene, and limit your intake of sugar, which leads to an overgrowth of acid-producing bacteria (good and bad).

RECOMMENDED PROBIOTIC REGIMEN

When suffering from a canker sore, it is best to take powdered probiotics, which begin working in the mouth immediately.

* Take ½ teaspoon each *L. acidophilus*, *B. bifidum*, and *L. bulgaricus* powders, mixed together in 6 to 8 ounces unchilled unfiltered water, three times daily before each meal. Before swallowing, swish the liquid in your mouth a few seconds.
* In addition to the above regimen, for increased strength, take 1 combination capsule that contains all three super strains in an oil-matrix carrier, once a day.

NOTE: For choosing the highest quality probiotics, see guidelines beginning on page 137.

Clostridium perfringens Poisoning

See Food Poisoning.

Cold Sores. *See also* Canker Sores; Dental Problems.

Cold sores, also known as fever blisters, are caused by herpes simplex virus I. Highly contagious, cold sores usually appear three to five days after exposure. Depending on their severity, they may last up to three weeks. The virus, which then remains in the body, can be triggered by fever, a cold or other viral infection, exposure to the sun, stress, or a depressed immune system. Usually appearing on the lips or the hard part of the gums, cold sores often begin as a tender bump, which soon turns into a blister or a cluster of blisters.

Keeping your friendly bacterial army strong is helpful in reducing the recurrence of cold sore outbreaks. (The antiviral capabilities of your beneficial bacteria are detailed in Chapter 8.)

RECOMMENDED PROBIOTIC REGIMEN

When suffering from cold sores, it is best to take powdered probiotics, which begin working in the mouth immediately. A strong probiotic regimen is recommended to subdue these herpes virus outbreaks.

- Take 1 teaspoon each *L. acidophilus, B. bifidum,* and *L. bulgaricus* powders, mixed together in 6 to 8 ounces chilled unfiltered water, three times daily before each meal. Before swallowing, swish the liquid in your mouth a few seconds.
- In addition to the above regimen, for increased strength, take 1 combination capsule that contains all three super strains in an oil-matrix carrier, once a day.

NOTE: For choosing the highest quality probiotics, see guidelines beginning on page 137.

Colitis.

See Ulcerative Colitis, Irritable Bowel Syndrome.

Constipation.

Waste material that moves through the large intestine too slowly results in constipation. Constipation can cause a number of ailments including bad breath, gas, nausea, fatigue, coated tongue, irritability, headaches, and abdominal cramps. Chronic constipation may be involved in the development of hemorrhoids, diverticulitis, and colon cancer. Because the intestines are a breeding ground for toxins, it is important that the "transit time" for waste material is no longer than twenty-four hours. After this time, antigens and toxins begin to breed.

At one time or another, most of us have experienced a bout with constipation. Although a change in bowel (or bladder) habits is one of the warning signs of cancer, an occasional difficult bowel movement is rarely reason for concern.

Often arising from a diet with too little fluid and fiber, constipation is the possible result of laxative overuse, a stomach or intestinal blockage, nerve or muscle damage, or weak intestinal muscles. Certain drugs, such as painkillers and antidepressants, and mineral supplements, such as iron, are also common suspects in causing constipation. Pregnancy is another common cause.

Another primary cause of constipation is too few friendly intestinal bacteria. The friendly bacteria are helpful in encouraging peristalsis—the rhythmic muscular activity that moves the contents of the intestines along. Peristalsis is more efficient when the acidity of the region increases, and that's where lactobacteria are helpful. As part of their normal fermentation process, lactobacteria produce lactic, acetic, and other acids, creating an environment that enhances peristalsis.

Several studies have shown the benefits of lactobacteria on chronic constipation resulting from a disturbed gastrointestinal tract. One study conducted by Drs. Rajala, et al., involved elderly hospitalized patients who suffered with constipation. The subjects were given yogurt that contained *L. acidophilus* supplemented with fiber and lactitol (a disaccharide alcohol that is food for *L. acidophilus*). This resulted in a significant reduction of constipation.

Another study conducted in Sweden by Livia Alm, et al., involved forty-two patients between the ages of fifty and ninety-five who suffered from chronic constipation. All had become dependent on various forms of laxatives. The patients were divided into two groups. The first group was given as much acidophilus milk at breakfast as they wanted for seven weeks. The other group received no fermented foods. After the initial seven weeks was up, the acidophilus milk was withdrawn from the first group. During the next six weeks, the members of the second group enjoyed acidophilus milk with their breakfasts. A log was kept showing how much acidophilus milk was consumed by each patient. Their bowel action and the consistency of their bowel movements were monitored as well. There was a marked reduction in the amount of laxatives needed and the degree of constipation during the periods in which the acidophilus milk was consumed; this was confirmed by the number and consistency of the subjects' bowel movements. The study determined that the best effect against chronic constipation was achieved with an intake of 200 milliliters (about six ounces) per day of acidophilus milk.

The elderly often suffer from chronic constipation for a number of reasons. Erratic or improper diet that leads to nutritional deficiencies, and lack of physical activity are the most common causes. Many have relied on laxatives for so long that their bodies no longer work on "automatic," but must rely on the stimulation of a laxative to initiate peristalsis. Then, too, an aging body slows down, and the bowels no longer work as they once did. The added bonus received by geriatric patients who eat cultured foods (or take probiotic supplements) is a dramatic improvement in nutritional intake, including practically predigested proteins and bioavailable calcium.

The friendly bacteria are helpful for anyone suffering from chronic constipation, not just the elderly. Taking probiotic supplements, eating real yogurt, or drinking sweet acidophilus milk offer great help without any negative side effects.

RECOMMENDED PROBIOTIC REGIMEN

When beginning a probiotic regimen to combat constipation, it is important to realize that, depending on the level of toxicity, the die-off of toxins may result in the Herxheimer Reaction—gas, bloating, and possible headaches (see inset on page 148). Depending on the discomfort level you are willing to handle, it may be best to start with minimal amounts of probiotics, gradually increasing their amount and frequency as you see fit. Powders are the recommended form.

- Start with ½ teaspoon each of *L. acidophilus*, *B. bifidum*, and *L. bulgaricus* powders mixed together in 6 to 8 ounces unchilled filtered water, taken three times daily before meals. Can increase the amounts to 1 teaspoon each *L acidophilus* and *B. bifidum powders*, and 1 tablespoon *L. bulgaricus*.

NOTE: For choosing the highest quality probiotics, see guidelines beginning on page 137.

Crohn's Disease.

Crohn's disease is a condition in which the immune system attacks its own cells, most commonly those that line sections of the walls of both the small and large intestines. This painful inflammation causes chronic diarrhea, abdominal cramping, fever, weight loss, and loss of appetite. It can lead to the development of bowel obstructions and abscesses. When the large intestine is affected, rectal bleeding is common; after prolonged periods, the risk of cancer is increased. Individuals who suffer from the most severe form of the disease are often unable to work or participate in normal activities.

This disabling bowel disorder affects as many as 500,000 Americans and is considered medically incurable. Although its cause is unknown, a weakened immune system, infection, and diet are the most common suspects. While a few people recover completely after a single attack of Crohn's disease, most find themselves experiencing regular flare-ups.

The favored treatments for Crohn's disease are steroids and antibiotics, but both are only marginally effective and sometimes cause severe side effects. Surgical removal of the most severely affected areas of the intestines is often the last resort, but even this is not a sure cure and symptoms inevitably return.

A 1996 research study at Cedars-Sinai Medical Center offers a small glimmer of hope for victims of Crohn's disease. It has been determined that the affected cells contain large quantities of cytokines (proteins) produced by the immune system. One such cytokine, called tumor necrosis factor (TNF), has been implicated in cancer and a variety of other diseases, as well as in Crohn's disease.

The scientists at Cedars-Sinai are using special antibodies (monoclonal) that bind specifically to TNF and remove it from the bloodstream. The theory is that removing this cytokine from the blood before it reaches the intestines may be the best hope of eliminating Crohn's disease. About 65 percent of the patients who received the anti-TNF antibodies showed a dramatic reduction of symptoms, while the remaining patients had no response. These results indicate that there may be several different cytokines that cause Crohn's disease. Currently, the research team is analyzing the cytokines in the patients who did not respond to the anti-TNF antibody in the hope of designing new antibodies that can target other cytokines.

In 1994, Dr. Michael L. McCann and colleagues published a paper entitled, "Recolonization Therapy with Nonadhesive *Escherichia coli* for Treatment of Inflammatory Bowel Disease," in the *Journal of the New York Academy of Sciences.* This work reported on a process called "reflorastation" and a three-year study that focused on normalizing the bowel bacteria using *L. acidophilus* (DDS-1 strain), *B. bifidum* (Malyoth strain), and benign *E. coli* bacteria (Nissel 1917 strain). Remember, *E. coli* is a common bowel bacteria that we all carry. With the exception of the lethal H:0157 strain, which contaminates the food chain, most strains of *E. coli* are harmless. Because they are normal bowel residents they can even be considered beneficial.

Dr. McCann's study involved patients who suffered from an inflammatory bowel disease, either Crohn's disease or ulcerative colitis. His reflorastation protocol began with the use of heavy-duty antibiotics and antifungals to completely rid the body of all bacteria—the good as well as the bad. Once the intestines had been thoroughly denuded, the normal bacteria were reintroduced, both orally and via retention enemas. As a result, each patient so treated went into remission, and those who continued with the bacterial supplementation remain disease-free at the time of this writing.

The paper concludes, "A subset of patients with inflammatory bowel disease who are successfully recolonized with nonadhesive *E. coli* [and the friendly bacteria] achieved complete, sustained, drug-free remissions. . . . Reflorastation is not only a method that has the potential to identify putative etiologic antigens, but is also a clinical method to induce long-term remissions without the use of toxic drugs."

RECOMMENDED PROBIOTIC REGIMEN

- Take ½ teaspoon *L. bulgaricus* powder mixed in 8 ounces unchilled filtered water, three times daily. May add ½ teaspoon each of *L. acidophilus* and *B. bifidum* powders (or 1 capsule each).

- In addition to the above regimen, for increased strength, take 1 combination capsule that contains all three super strains in an oil-matrix carrier, two to three times daily.

NOTE: For choosing the highest quality probiotics, see guidelines beginning on page 137.

Dental Problems. *See also* Mouth Sores.

As explained in Chapter 2, digestion begins in your mouth where the enzymes in saliva begin to digest carbohydrates. The environment in your mouth is meant to be slightly alkaline, not acidic. However, a diet rich in sugar coupled with poor oral hygiene disturbs the pH balance and the mouth becomes a breeding ground for acid-loving, acid-producing bacteria. Sugar provides the food for these bacteria, and the acid they produce becomes the "glue" of dental plaque—the cement-like substance that must be scraped off your teeth.

The primary suspect in dental disease is *Streptococcus mutans* and other streptococcal strains, as well as *Candida albicans*. However, certain friendly strains of *Lactobacillus, L. casei,* and bifidobacteria are also implicated. How does it happen that these friends turn foe? You see, as a rule, lactobacilli are not a primary cause in the formation of dental caries. Rather they are the normal beneficial flora of the mouth and account for only 0.01 percent of the bacteria responsible for plaque. However, quantities of lactobacilli have been found to increase in a small number of cases in which dental decay has already begun. In other words, these friendly bacteria are secondary contributors to tooth decay—they turn foe only once the trouble has started. Therefore, it is safe to assume that beneficial lactobacilli are not involved in causing cavities.

Take a situation in which beneficial bacteria can flourish in a region of the body where they are not normal colonizers, such as the mouth. Under ideal circumstances, the natural flora of the mouth—including the right strains of the friendly bacteria—provide a barrier to canker sores and dental decay. For example, lactobacilli fight oral yeasts, such as the *Candida albicans* bacteria that may contribute to dental decay. To inhibit the action of every kind of bacteria that attack teeth, protect the normal alkaline environment of your mouth by limiting the sugar in your diet, which leads to an overgrowth of acid-producing bacteria (good and bad), and by practicing good oral hygiene.

RECOMMENDED PROBIOTIC REGIMEN

- Take ½ teaspoon each of *L. acidophilus, B. bifidum* and *L. bulgaricus* powders, mixed together in 6 to 8 ounces unchilled filtered water,

one to three times daily before meals. Before swallowing, swish the
liquid in your mouth a few seconds.

- Instead of the above regimen, take 1 combination capsule that contains all three super strains in an oil-matrix carrier, one to three
times daily.

NOTE: For choosing the highest quality probiotics, see guidelines beginning on page 137.

Depression. *See also* Anxiety; Stress.

A feeling of intense sadness, depression is an illness that encompass-
es the entire person— physical body, moods, thoughts, and behavior.
Varying in severity and persistence, depression can last for days or
years. Typically, people who are depressed tend to lose interest in the
world around them and are incapable of experiencing happiness.
Common symptoms include insomnia or the need for excessive sleep,
loss of or increase in appetite, restlessness, irritability, digestive disorders, apathy, sadness, and feelings of worthlessness.

Causes of depression may include emotionally upsetting events,
side effects of certain medications, poor diet, and intense stress.
Heredity is another significant factor. Other possible causes include
physical illness, nutritional deficiencies, and food allergies.

We think primarily of a patient's mental state when the diagnosis
is an anxiety disorder or depression. Nonetheless, the friendly bacteria may be of some help in alleviating these conditions if they are used
as part of a comprehensive, therapeutic treatment plan. Several medical experts have suggested that supplemental lactobacteria can help
in those patients suffering from anxiety and depression.

In their 1984 paper, "Nutritional and Therapeutic Aspects of Lactobacilli," published in the *Journal of Applied Nutrition,* Drs. B.A.
Friend and K.M. Shahani wrote, "While there are no direct data
relating lactobacilli to the alleviation of anxiety and depressive
symptoms, indirect evidence suggests a possible relationship . . . lactobacilli release essential amino acids during fermentation, and fermented dairy products are rich in several essential amino acids,
including tryptophan."

Your body uses tryptophan to produce serotonin—a neurotransmitter with a calming effect. If you've ever had a cup of warm milk at night to help you relax and sleep, you should know that it is the tryptophan in milk that makes this traditional insomnia remedy work. The action of the friendly bacteria in a cultured milk product, such as yogurt, results in even more tryptophan, which, in turn, means more relaxing serotonin. Because the bacteria are so densely concentrated in quality probiotics, it's easy to see that taking supplemental lactobacteria may work best of all.

In his paper, "Lactobacilli and Human Health," Dr. C.S. Hangee-Bauer notes that patients who are suffering from anxiety and depression might well prove to be deficient in beneficial bacteria. He reminds us that toxic causes are implicated in some mental aberrations, and, "Colonization of the intestines with lactobacilli reduces the amounts of endotoxins produced by certain bacteria, some of which have been linked with a wide variety of inflammatory and mental disorders."

Serious cases of anxiety and depression require the prompt attention of an expert mental health professional. These are not problems for simple self-care. However, there is clear evidence that toxins produced by harmful bacteria, as well as a nutritional deficiency or imbalance, can contribute to a depressed mental state.

Keeping your armies of friendly bacteria strong can help in the inhibition of harmful bacteria and other toxic microorganisms. Furthermore, lactobacilli's capability of producing tryptophan, which stimulates mood relaxing seratonin can be helpful in creating a calm mood. Remember, probiotics are not only eminently beneficial, they are perfectly safe. The friendly bacteria perform so many useful services for your body that there's no reason not to take probiotics daily, especially in cases of anxiety and depression. Remember, friendly bacteria cannot hurt, they can only help in eliciting a sense of calmness and clarity.

RECOMMENDED PROBIOTIC REGIMEN

- Take 1 capsule each of *L. acidophilus* and *B. bifidum* (or ½ teaspoon each powder), along with ½ teaspoon *L. bulgaricus* powder mixed in 6 to 8 ounces unchilled filtered water, three times daily. Take 10 to 30 minutes before meals.

- Instead of the above regimen, take 1 or 2 combination capsules that contain all three super strains in an oil-matrix carrier, once a day.

NOTE: For choosing the highest quality probiotics, see guidelines beginning on page 137.

Diabetes Mellitus.

Diabetes mellitus results from inadequate insulin production by the pancreas. Insulin is necessary for the body to utilize glucose—blood sugar. It allows glucose to be transported into cells so they can produce energy. After eating or drinking, the rise in blood sugar stimulates the pancreas to produce insulin. When the body doesn't produce enough insulin to maintain normal blood sugar levels, diabetes is the result.

There are two kinds of diabetes mellitus—type I and type II. Those with type I diabetes, also known as juvenile diabetes, produce little or no insulin at all, due to the destruction of the insulin-producing cells in the pancreas. Symptoms include frequent urination, unusual thirst, weight loss despite normal intake of food, and nausea and/or vomiting. In type II or adult-onset diabetes, the pancreas continues to produce insulin, however, the body doesn't utilize it. Common symptoms include unusual thirst, fatigue, skin infections, frequent urination, slow wound healing, tingling feet, and blurry vision. Type II diabetes is often linked to a poor diet.

Overgrowth of the harmful *Escherichia coli* bacteria is linked to diabetes. In 1981, the *Journal of Biological Chemistry* published a paper entitled, "Insulin or a Closely Related Molecule is Native to *E. coli*," by Drs. D. LeRoith, J. Shiloach, J. Roth, and M. Lesniak. The scientists revealed evidence that certain strains of this common bowel bacteria produce a substance the body cannot distinguish from insulin. Insulin, of course, is what controls the levels of sugar in the blood.

The research team found that some people suffering from adult-onset diabetes had what seemed to be normal levels of insulin in their blood, but it wasn't working as it should. They discovered that the pseudo-insulin produced by *E. coli* may block special receptor sites on cells that insulin must reach in order to control blood sugar levels. When the body's own insulin is blocked by the insulin-like substance produced by certain strains of *E. coli*, sugar levels in the blood can rise, resulting in a diabetic condition.

It is, therefore, important to keep these strains of *E. coli* bacteria from breeding. Avoid high-fat and high-sugar diets, which encourage the decline of bifidobacteria and the dramatic rise of bacteria such as *E. coli*.

RECOMMENDED PROBIOTIC REGIMEN

- Take 1 capsule each of *L. acidophilus* and *B. bifidum* (or ½ teaspoon each powder), along with ½ teaspoon *L. bulgaricus* powder mixed in 6 to 8 ounces unchilled filtered water, three times daily. Take 10 to 30 minutes before meals.
- Instead of the above regimen, take 1 or 2 combination capsules that contain all three super strains in an oil-matrix carrier, once a day.

NOTE: For choosing the highest quality probiotics, see guidelines beginning on page 137.

Diaper Rash.

The common diaper rash is an inflammation of the skin that is caused by a reaction to the enzymes and chemicals in the urine and feces, as well as to the perfumes and chemicals in some soaps and lotions. Often areas of the skin are swollen and sometimes dry and scaly. A fungal diaper rash, which is caused by an overgrowth of *Candida albicans* in the intestinal tract, results in smooth, shiny skin, that is bright red in color. The borders of the rash are well defined, and there may be scattered spots in the groin area.

As seen in Chapter 5, "Babies and Friendly Bacteria," the way in which your baby was born—vaginally or by cesarean section—strongly influences the type of bacteria your infant will carry in his or her intestinal tract. Babies pick up friendly (or unfriendly) bacteria from their mothers as they pass through the birth canal. If the baby's intestinal tract is overrun with harmful bacteria or a yeast/fungus like *Candida albicans,* he or she will be susceptible to a number of problems, including chronic diaper rash. (Remember, the skin is a secondary exit route for those toxins in the body that are not excreted via the urine or feces.)

In addition to treating the child's rash with a topical probiotic paste, it is very important to build up the friendly bacteria in his or her gastrointestinal tract. Treating the rash only, without taking care of the internal flora, will result in a temporary solution at best. Remember, health begins on the inside.

RECOMMENDED PROBIOTIC REGIMEN

- Mix ¼ teaspoon *B. infantis* powder in the baby's formula at each feeding. (You can also mix the powder in juice or water and administer it to your child in an eye dropper.) If breastfeeding, mix the same amount of *B. infantis* in a little water and apply it to your nipple area as the baby feeds. Once the rash has disappeared, it is prudent to continue this regimen until the child has been introduced to solid foods or until age two.

- Prepare a topical application by mixing 1 teaspoon *L. bulgaricus* or *L. acidophilus* powder with enough water or probiotic face cream (page 202) to form a smooth paste. After cleansing the area, gently pat it dry with a clean towel and apply the paste generously to the inflamed area(s). Cover loosely (or leave the diaper off completely) and allow the paste to dry. During each diaper change, reapply the paste to any areas where needed. Also reapply the paste each time the area is washed. At night, cover the area with a thick layer of pure pharmaceutical lanolin. Be generous with this "covering," which will serve as a shield against any urine or feces in the nighttime diaper. Apply the lanolin as you would a thick layer of frosting.

- Once the diaper rash has cleared and the skin is back to normal, continue applying the lanolin or face cream to the area for at least two weeks to prevent recurrence. (The best strategy is to continue applying the lanolin or face cream to the baby's bottom until he or she is out of diapers.)

NOTE: For choosing the highest quality probiotics, see guidelines beginning on page 137.

Diarrhea.

Diarrhea is characterized by excessive and frequent bowel movements that are loose and watery. Accompanying symptoms might include abdominal pain and cramping, fever, thirst, and vomiting. Excessive or prolonged diarrhea can cause dehydration due to the water loss from the body. It can interfere with nutrient absorption because the digested food rushes through the intestines before nutrients can be extracted and absorbed. Diarrhea can also throw your body's pH level off balance.

Diarrhea can be the result of a number of causes, including the ingestion of certain foods, lactose intolerance, food poisoning, the side effects of certain drugs, infection, inflammation, irritation, influenza, and poisonous toxins produced by invading pathogenic bacteria. More serious causes for diarrhea include intestinal tumors and malabsorption syndrome—a condition in which the intestines cannot efficiently absorb the nutrients in foods.

No matter what the cause, when you suffer from diarrhea, you lose vast numbers of bacteria at a very fast rate in a very short period of time. This condition dramatically and quickly affects the friendly bacterial populations of the bowel. At times, the resident beneficial bacteria can be completely overwhelmed by the activities of an invading pathogen—bacterial or viral—that produces diarrhea by its toxic byproducts.

What happens in the large intestine differs when the pathogenic invader is a bacterial colonizer (such as *Salmonella, Shigella,* and *E. coli*) or a transient bacteria (including *Staphylococcus aureus,* some strains of *Clostridium,* and *Bacillus cereus).* Obviously, any bacterial strain that aims to take up residence is more difficult to deal with than one that will pass through naturally in time. The diarrhea itself can be the result of the rapid growth of colonizing harmful bacteria, or the toxins that both colonizers and transients produce.

Whatever medical treatment your doctor may recommend to deal with acute diarrhea, and that depends on the root cause, your first responsibility is to promptly replace the friendly bacteria you have lost. When you reinforce the friendly bacteria with effective probiotics, no matter what the cause of your diarrhea might be, you are giving your body what it needs to restore health to the region.

RECOMMENDED PROBIOTIC REGIMEN

- Take ½ teaspoon each of *L. acidophilus*, *B. bifidum* powders, (or 1 capsule each), along with ½ teaspoon *L. bulgaricus* powder mixed in 6 to 8 ounces unchilled filtered water. Continue this regimen every hour until symptoms subside.

NOTE: For choosing the highest quality probiotics, see guidelines beginning on page 137.

Dry skin.

See Skin Problems.

Escherichia coli (E. coli) Poisoning.

See Food Poisoning.

Fever Blisters.

See Cold Sores.

Food Poisoning.

When a person eats food that is infected with harmful microorganisms (usually bacteria), the result is food poisoning. If you have ever suffered an upset stomach accompanied by a bout of diarrhea after a meal, you may have eaten something that disagreed with you. Nausea, upset stomach, and accompanying diarrhea are the classic symptoms of mild food poisoning.

According to the latest data, food poisoning affects up to 80 million persons every year in the United States alone. It has been estimated that as many 9,000 people die annually in this country from foodborne infections. The problem is serious, and it's not going away. In fact, it's on the rise.

TYPES OF FOOD POISONING

According to the United States Centers for Disease Control (CDC), more than 250 foodborne diseases have been identified. Symptoms of these diseases vary widely, depending on the infectious agent. The most common types of bacterial food poisoning are salmonellosis, *Staphylococcus aureus* poisoning, botulism, *Clostridium perfringens* poisoning, *Escherichia coli* (*E. coli*) poisoning, and listeriosis.

Salmonellosis

Salmonella bacteria are part of the intestinal flora found in a number of animals. Easily transmitted through improper food handling, salmonella is the leading cause of food poisoning and death in the United States. Over half the livestock—cows, poultry, and pigs—are given antibiotics to protect them from the infectious agents that dwell in their crowded, unsanitary environments. *Salmonella* bacteria thrive in animals that have been given antibiotics.

Symptoms of *Salmonella* poisoning (salmonellosis), which usually develop within eight to thirty-six hours after eating contaminated food, include fever, chills, nausea, vomiting, abdominal cramps, diarrhea, and general discomfort. Eggs and chickens are the most common sources of *Salmonella* bacteria, although beef, pork, contaminated milk, raw clams and oysters, as well as sushi made from raw fish are culprits as well.

Approximately 25 percent of all chickens sold in the United States are contaminated with *Salmonella*, and up to 90 percent of all chickens carry harmful *Campylobacter* bacteria, now known as *Helicobacter pylori*. Eggs are not safe, either. In fact, about 80 percent of all meat- and poultry-related illnesses, and 75 percent of the resulting deaths, are caused by one of these two bacteria that are commonly found in poultry and eggs. Those who eat raw or incompletely cooked meats and eggs are at even greater risk of *Salmonella* poisoning.

Common symptoms of salmonellosis can range from mild abdominal cramps and vomiting to severe diarrhea and high fever. Dehydration is a concern. According to the latest data, salmonella kills more than 4,000 Americans annually and sickens as many as 5 million every year. Medical costs and lost wages due to salmonellosis are estimated to be more than $1 billion per year.

Finally, in March of 1998, came a significant breakthrough in the use of probiotics in the war against salmonellosis. The Food and Drug Administration approved the use of Preempt—a culture of 29 friendly bacteria that can help prevent *Salmonella* contamination in chickens. The technique involves spraying newborn chicks with the solution of these friendly bacteria. As the chicks peck at their feathers, they ingest the bacterial solution. The friendly bacteria then take up residence in their intestinal tracts, preventing harmful microbes from proliferating. During the FDA trials, the *Salmonella* contamination in chickens was reduced to zero. Furthermore, at this point, although the FDA approval is for control only of *Salmonella* in chickens, tests have indicated success against other food-poisoning bacteria such as *Campylobacter* and *Listeria*.

Escherichia coli Poisoning

There are hundreds of strains of *Escherichia coli (E. coli)* bacteria. Most live in the intestines of healthy people and animals. For the most part, they pose no problems. However, the 0157:H7 strain, first identified in 1982, can be deadly. This strain, which causes hemorrhagic colitis, is showing up throughout the world in increasing numbers.

Persons infected with this strain of *E. coli* characteristically develop sudden, extremely painful abdominal cramps and severe, watery diarrhea that typically becomes bloody within twenty-four hours. For most, the illness subsides in five to ten days. If, however, the *E. coli* toxins permeate the intestinal wall and are absorbed into the bloodstream, they can cause hemolytic uremic syndrome (HUS), which can cause kidney failure. Other possible complications include seizure and stroke.

Major sources of the 0157:H7 strain include undercooked beef, especially ground beef, and raw milk. Bacteria lurking in a cow's udders or in milking equipment that has been inadequately sterilized can be passed into the raw milk. Fortunately, the pasteurization process kills this bacteria.

If the 0157:H7 bacterial strain has invaded the intestines of cattle during the slaughtering process, it can contaminate meat that is sold to the consumer. Know that one small contaminated section of beef can infect many pounds of ground beef. Although *E. coli* bacteria are destroyed when ground meat is thoroughly cooked, they live on in a rare, juicy hamburger.

Water-borne transmission of 0157:H7 has also been documented, but chlorinated (or carbonated) water is generally considered safe. Because *E. coli* 0157:H7 can pass from person to person, especially among children in diapers, it is a major concern for day-care center operators. Frequent handwashing with antibacterial soap will prevent transmission.

Staphylococcus aureus Poisoning

Food contaminated with the toxins produced by *Staphylococcus aureus* bacteria make up 25 percent of all food poisoning cases. The contamination typically occurs when a food handler with a staphylococcal skin infection touches food that is left to sit out at room temperature. This enables the bacteria to proliferate and produce toxins. As the staphylococci microorganism is typically found in the nose and throat, a food can also become contaminated if it is sneezed or coughed on.

Symptoms, which typically begin suddenly within two to eight hours after the contaminated food is eaten, include severe nausea and vomiting. Cramping, diarrhea, headache, and fever are other common symptoms. Staphylococcal toxin typically contaminates cream-filled pastries; milk and milk products; tuna, potato, and macaroni salads; meats (especially processed varieties); and fish. (For additional information on *S. aureus* bacteria, see the inset on page 208.)

Listeriosis

Listeria bacteria infects shellfish, birds, spiders, and mammals (including cows) in all areas of the world. It is transmitted to humans by direct contact with infected animals or their secretions, by breathing infected dust, or through contact with contaminated sewage or soil. All secretions from an infected person or animal may contain the organism. Listeriosis is most commonly transmitted through the consumption of contaminated dairy products or raw vegetables.

Signs of listeriosis, which occur two to four weeks after exposure to the organism, include shock, heart inflammation, enlarged liver and spleen, and circulatory collapse. A dark red rash may spread over the trunk and legs. The signs and severity of the disease vary according to the site of infection and the age and condition of the patient. In adults, the most common form of listeriosis is meningitis (infection of the membranes covering the brain and the spinal cord). Left untreated, meningitis can result in coma and death. Those with weakened immune systems, newborns, and those over seventy years old are most susceptible to listeriosis. It is especially serious in pregnant women, and fetal infection transmitted through the placenta is usually fatal to the child. About 30 percent of those infected with *Listeria* die.

Botulism

Life-threatening, foodborne botulism is caused by highly poisonous toxins produced by the *Clostridium botulinum* bacteria. One of the most serious of the various types of food poisoning, botulism affects the central nervous system.

What makes this food poisoning different from most others is that it develops without stomach upset. Nausea and vomiting occur in less than half the cases. After eating contaminated food, symptoms can begin suddenly anywhere from four hours to eight days, with early symptoms that include double vision, droopy eyelids, sensitivity to light, the inability to focus on an object, and difficulty in swallowing. Muscle weakness eventually affects the entire body, and may result in respiratory failure, paralysis, and even death.

The most common botulism sources include improperly cooked or canned vegetables, fish, fruits, and condiments. Beef, pork, poultry, and milk products are also common suspects. Home-canned foods are the most common source, although commercially prepared foods can be responsible as well. This is due to improper canning techniques, usually inadequate sealing. Beware of cans with bulging lids and jars with cracks—true signs that the food within may be contaminated.

(Botulism can occur in containers with no signs of damage, as well.) Foods that are kept at room temperature for prolonged periods of time, as in some cafeterias and delis, can provide the proper environment for the growth of *Clostridium botulinum*. Heating food to a temperature of at least 176°F destroys most of the poisonous bacteria.

Clostridium perfringens Poisoning

Foods, especially meat and meat products, that are contaminated with toxins produced by *Clostridium perfringens* bacteria result in gastroenteritis. Some strains of the bacteria produce toxins that cause mild bouts of nausea and vomiting that generally last less than a day. Other strains can cause severe episodes that are characterized by strong abdominal pain and vomiting, bloody diarrhea, abdominal distention from gas, and dehydration. Severe cases can cause intestinal holes, severe loss of body fluids, poisoning of the bowel area (peritonitis), and/or blood poisoning (septicemia).

Most *Clostridium perfringens* toxins are heat-resistant and not affected by normal cooking. The bacteria multiply, form spores, and create toxins that multiply as foods cool.

GOVERNMENTAL ACTION

Due to the growing number of food poisoning incidents (see The Growing Problem of Food Poisoning, beginning on page 178), the government has started taking action in an attempt to better protect the public.

New regulations governing the meat and poultry industries are already in place. In July 1996, President Bill Clinton signed a bill requiring producers to reduce the acceptable levels of bacteria in their meat and poultry. This may not seem like an improvement, but it is. Under the existing regulations, which were established in 1907, inspectors rely on "sniff and poke" tests to detect unsafe meat and poultry. However, until putrefaction sets in, most bacteria don't give themselves away.

The new procedures will feature scientific testing for bacterial contamination. Individual companies have up to forty-two months to establish their "hazard control" systems, and the meat and poultry processors themselves will test for *E. coli*. Federal inspectors will conduct spot tests for *Salmonella* at various stages of production. While

The Growing Problem of Food Poisoning

Food poisoning is often mistaken for the flu. You have undoubtedly experienced a mild case yourself—few of us escape it. However, headlines of serious outbreaks are becoming more frequent and universal. It seems that almost every day we read or hear of a problem with food poisoning in some area of the world, with more and more of these episodes occurring in the United States.

In 1985, over 17,000 people in Illinois were poisoned by *Salmonella typhimurium*, and 14 died. The source of this food poisoning epidemic was contaminated milk. It was discovered that during the bottling process, contaminated raw milk had been mixed accidentally with milk that had already been pasteurized.

In the United States, the largest outbreak of food poisoning recorded to date occurred in 1994, when 3.4 million people in forty different states ate ice cream that was contaminated with salmonella from unpasteurized eggs. The ice cream itself hadn't been made with unpasteurized eggs, but the tanker truck that transported the ice cream premix to the manufacturer had previously contained unpasteurized liquid eggs that had been contaminated with salmonella. The tankers were supposed to have been thoroughly cleaned before they were filled with the ice cream premix, but inspectors found that several tankers had not been cleaned adequately. They also discovered cracks in the lining of at least five of the trucks.

According to the *New England Journal of Medicine*, of the 3.4 million people who ate the contaminated ice cream, 224,000 of them suffered from *salmonella enteriditis*, a form of food poisoning that causes fever, chills, and bloody diarrhea.

Do you take mayonnaise-dressed salads to a picnic or a potluck meal? Be aware that they must be kept cold—under 40°F. In 1975, at a community picnic, 139 people fell ill after eating contaminated potato salad. The cause was *Haemolytic streptococcus*, confirmed by throat cultures of sixty-three of the sick picnickers.

Another member of the streptococcus family—a gastrointestinal bacteria called *enterococcus*—has been raising havoc recently. Most enterococci are harmless, but one particular strain has begun to mutate out of the reach of every drug, even vancomycin—the "biggest gun" in the antibiotic arsenal that, until recently, was considered the never-fail antibiotic. Because of its resistance to vancomycin, this harmful strain of enterococci has been named VRE, which stands for vancomycin-resistant enterococcus.

VRE is usually found in contaminated microscopic fecal matter. The bacteria spreads easily because of its ability to live for days on surfaces like kitchen countertops. Those most at risk of VRE poisoning are the very young, the very old, the very ill, and those with compromised immune systems. This is why patients in hospitals, skilled nursing facilities, and nursing homes face a greater risk of VRE than most others.

In February 1994, an outbreak of VRE in Los Angeles sickened thirty-one people. Within six months, half of them were dead. Every state in the nation has reported cases of VRE, but the majority have been found in the northeastern United States. Nonetheless, this is a coast-to-coast problem. Hospitals in New York and California have confirmed treating VRE outbreaks involving dozens of patients.

In Massachusetts in 1983, forty-nine people were hospitalized with septicemia (blood poisoning) or meningitis (an infection of the membranes surrounding the brain and spinal cord). Fourteen of the patients died. The root cause of both of these diseases was traced to Listeria monocytogenes, which was found in a particular brand of milk. At the same time, another incident occurred in Connecticut, and the same milk source was at fault. After a thorough investigation, it was discovered that the dairy cows that provided this milk had had mastitis and were infected with Listeria. The puzzling question was how the Listeria survived the pasteurization process, which had been done properly according to the investigators.

Recently, a number of outbreaks of Listeria food poisoning have been linked to pasteurized cheeses, and various studies have also identified this bacteria in pasteurized nonfat milk and cottage cheese. It seems frighteningly clear that standard pasteurization procedures are not capable of destroying the Listeria bacteria. This is very worrisome in light of the fact that, in some tests, as much as 12 percent of all raw milk in the United States has been found to be contaminated with Listeria bacteria.

The spring and summer of 1996 saw an outbreak of food poisoning that reportedly sickened more than 1,000 people in eleven different states. Cyclospora, an intestinal microorganism that causes intense diarrhea, weight loss, and extreme fatigue, was identified as the source. Although raspberries and strawberries were investigated as possible sources, the tests were inconclusive. Identifying the source of contamination is difficult because Cyclospora has an incubation period of seven days, and often several more days pass before the case is reported. By then, according to the CDC, memories are hazy and trying to track the course of the disease is difficult. The long incubation period and delays in arriving at the correct diagnosis have complicated the problem. Many labs do not test for Cyclospora, and workers are not adequately trained to detect it.

The deadly E. coli strain 0157:H7 kills about 400 people every year and sickens another 20,000. In 1993, an episode of food poisoning occurred in the Pacific Northwest that sickened upwards of 500 people and caused the death of several children. The outbreak was traced to undercooked fast-food hamburgers, but the initial source of the infected meat was never identified. According to C.T. Foreman, former Assistant Secretary of Agriculture, a single frozen hamburger patty can contain meat from dozens of animals, and some of the meat is likely to have come from meat producers in several different countries. In a case like this one, it is impossible to track down the true source of the contamination.

This same lethal E. coli strain has also sickened thousands of Japanese. All told, 9,412 cases of 0157:H7 were documented in Japan in 1996 and 1997. As of this writing, 319 of these people remain hospitalized, and eleven deaths have been recorded. Although radish sprouts were targeted as a likely cause of this bacterial contamination, even the most thorough testing has not implicated the sprouts as the source. The investigation is continuing.

The Federal Food & Drug Administration (FDA) claims that anywhere from 20,000 to 60,000 cases of food poisoning caused by tainted fish and shellfish occur every year in the United States. Shellfish are the culprits in more than 65 percent of all cases of food poisoning caused by seafood. Since May 1993, sixteen cases of infection by the bacteria Vibrio vulnificus have been documented in the Southwest. Raw oysters were the cause in each case. Half of those people infected with the bacteria died as a result.

A long-term examination of our use of pesticides, antibiotics, and other chemicals, and their connections to the spread of newly evolved deadly bacterial strains needs to be heightened and accelerated. The use of probiotics in soil, water, animals, and humans needs to be implemented. Stricter inspection standards are definitely in order to help protect consumers against tainted food products. Luckily, some governmental actions have been taken that will, hopefully, at least begin to eradicate this frightening problem (see page 177).

this is certainly a step in the right direction, spot-checking also means that not all beef and not all chickens will be tested for bacterial contamination, and nothing has been said about regulating egg producers.

The CDC reports that large numbers of *Salmonella* poisonings can be traced to contaminated eggs. Once *Salmonella* was transferred to eggshells as they came into contact with contaminated feces; however, today's modern farming methods insure that the shells are clean. Now, the *Salmonella* bacteria is actually inside the eggs. CDC tests indicate that chickens are contaminated internally, in the oviducts where eggs are formed. Even worse, factory-farmed chickens are regularly dosed with antibiotics. As a result, the *Salmonella* bacteria inside the eggs are likely to be resistant to most antibiotics. The good news, as mentioned in the section on Salmonellosis (page 173), is that the FDA has addressed this issue with the approval of the use of probiotics in a multibacterial spray called Preempt.

Preempt is a true step in the eradication of *Salmonella* contamination in chickens. Building up their intestinal linings with beneficial bacteria will prevent harmful salmonellosis from taking up residence there. Not only does this use of probiotics address the problem at its root, it also forces the elimination of antibiotic use in chickens. (Preempt and antibiotics cannot be used together, as the antibiotics kill the good bacteria.)

Currently, the government is also working on new laws to protect consumers from contaminated fish and shellfish. Under the old rules, the FDA set permissible levels of residue in shellfish, and individual states were responsible for enforcement. The new provisions will hold the manufacturers responsible for insuring that the fish they sell to consumers have been taken from approved waters and do not carry dangerous bacterial contaminants. At the time of this writing, these new regulations are still under discussion. Once they are signed into law, suppliers will presumably be given months, even years, to comply.

A FINAL WARNING

Unless it is organically produced, most of the meat or poultry in your supermarket comes from a factory farm where the animals have been given antibiotics from the time they were in their mother's womb until they are slaughtered. This means that the pathogenic bacteria they carry are very powerful. While the antibiotics may have been able to kill weaker bacterial strains, the super strains have survived the drugs.

When you come down with a case of food poisoning after eating bacterially contaminated food, you are getting a megadose of drug-resistant bacteria. With the advent of VRE (vancomycin-resistant enterococcus)—harmful bacteria that are resistant to vancomycin, the "biggest gun" in the antibiotic arsenal—the day has already arrived when even the most powerful broad-spectrum antibiotics may not be enough to destroy toxic foodborne pathogens.

Although antibiotics are often prescribed to treat most foodborne infections by killing the harmful bacteria, don't forget that they kill the important friendly bacteria as well. This permits the growth of certain harmful bacteria and other microorganisms that are resistant to antibiotics.

The best form of health insurance is the one provided by Nature. Probiotic supplements are the best way to keep your resident bacterial colonies healthy, active, and working on your behalf. Remember, the friendly bacteria are your first line of defense against food poisoning, even those potentially lethal foodborne infections.

RECOMMENDED PROBIOTIC REGIMEN

Remember, bouts of food poisoning are serious and require immediate medical attention. Nevertheless, you should begin taking probiotics before and after seeing your doctor. It is best to take powdered varieties—rather than capsules—when experiencing the nausea and diarrhea that generally accompany food poisoning. Continually taking small sips will help get these beneficial bacteria into the stomach quickly to help wash out the poisons.

- When experiencing food poisoning, mix 1 heaping teaspoon each of *L. acidophilus*, *B. bifidum*, and *L. bulgaricus* powders in 8 to 16 ounces unchilled filtered water. Take slow, small sips of this probiotic mixture through a straw every minute or so. When finished, repeat the procedure. Do this at least 3 times.
- When the episode is over and you're feeling better, take 1 capsule each of *L. acidophilus* and *B. bifidum* (or ½ teaspoon each powder), along with ½ teaspoon *L. bulgaricus* powder mixed in 6 to 8 ounces unchilled filtered water, two to three times daily for 1 month. To this regimen, you may also add or substitute 1 to 3 combination capsules that contain all three super strains in an oil-matrix carrier, daily.

NOTE: For choosing the highest quality probiotics, see guidelines beginning on page 137.

Protecting Yourself from Food Poisoning

There are many things that you can do to avoid becoming a victim of food poisoning. Here are some of them:

- *Always wash your hands before handling food.*
- *Whenever possible, purchase organically raised, antibiotic-free meat and poultry. Animals raised on factory farms are not only continually fed antibiotics, they are raised in crowded, unsanitary environments that encourage bacterial contamination.*
- *When you bring raw meat, poultry, or fish home from the supermarket, refrigerate it immediately (or freeze it for long-term storage). This will slow down bacterial growth.*
- *Defrost frozen meat, chicken, and fish in the refrigerator, not on*

kitchen countertops. Defrosting at room temperature encourages bacterial growth.

- *Never place cooked chicken, burgers, steaks, etc. on the same unwashed plate that held them raw. Always thoroughly wash the plate with hot soapy water first.*

- *When cutting raw chicken or turkey, never use the same knife or cutting board to also cut up vegetables or other foods without scrupulously disinfecting them first.*

- *After any contact with raw meat, poultry, or fish, always thoroughly disinfect your hands, kitchen countertops, cutting boards, and utensils with hot water and antibacterial soap immediately.*

- *Don't use the sauce in which raw chicken, meat, or fish has been marinating (unless it has been brought to a rolling boil for at least 1 minute.)*

- *Cook meat, poultry, and fish thoroughly and eat it as soon after cooking as possible. The center of any cooked meat must reach 165°F in order to kill bacteria. When cooking a roast, use a food thermometer to make sure the interior portion of the meat reaches this temperature. Burgers, steaks, chicken, and chops should be cooked until they are well done and no pink remains.*

- *Never allow any cooked food to stand out any longer than it takes to serve and eat it. Refrigerate leftovers as soon as possible. Grandmother used to allow the leftover roast or turkey to cool down before refrigerating it, but to avoid giving bacteria time to multiply, refrigerate food promptly.*

- *Keep the temperature of your refrigerator at 40°F or lower. Set your freezer to 0°F or lower.*

- *Don't use raw eggs that are cracked. They may contain a double-dose of antibiotic-resistant Salmonella or worse. When cooking eggs, aim for well-done. Boil eggs for seven minutes, poach for at least five minutes, and forget about "sunny side up" and "over easy." When frying eggs, it takes three minutes on each side before bacteria are destroyed. Always eat "dry" scrambled eggs.*

- *Wash produce thoroughly. Fruits, especially berries, and salad greens, such as leafy lettuces and spinach, often harbor contaminants. Never eat such foods until they are washed well.*

- *Be suspicious of products in damaged or bulging cans, cracked jars, or containers with loose lids. The contents of such items may be contaminated with Botulinum, the most dangerous of all foodborne bacteria. Throw them away. That tell-tale bulging can is the result of bacterial-produced gas and is letting you know that harmful bacteria are at work inside.*

- *If a just-opened can or jar of food is obviously moldy or smells wrong, throw it away; be suspicious of bubbles or foaminess. In all cases of suspected bacterial contamination, be sure to dispose of the food and container safely.*

- *Stay away from foods, especially those made with mayonnaise, salad dressing, and milk products, that have been unrefrigerated for more than an hour or two. Be especially leery of such items at picnics or potluck meals.*

- *When eating at salad bars, avoid those that don't look clean or those that are not covered by protective glass. Do not choose items such as chicken and fish, or foods containing mayonnaise.*

Even if you follow all of the safety precautions suggested above, your best bet for avoiding the serious consequences of food poisoning is to make sure the friendly bacteria are well represented in your gastrointestinal tract. Although laboratory-created antibiotics are no longer as effective as they once were, the powerful natural antibiotic weapons wielded by the friendly bacteria are as potent and powerful as always against invading bacteria.

Tips for Travelers

In most places, especially in Europe, those who are dining out order bottles of mineral water (sparkling and still) for the table as routinely as they select the wine for each course. I have observed that only Americans are satisfied with local water from the tap, and that's asking for trouble, for tap water is characteristically a breeding ground for bacteria and other microorganisms.

To minimize your risk of picking up unfriendly bacteria when traveling out of your local environment, follow these simple rules:

- *Drink only bottled water.*
- *Eat only fruit that you can peel (and personally peel it yourself).*
- *Eat only cooked foods.*
- *Eat only meats that have been cooked to the well-done stage.*
- *Don't eat anything from street vendors.*

Unless I am dining in a private home and know that the standards of my host are as high as mine, I even give up salads, although I love the crunch of crisp, raw greens. If dirty fingers have torn the lettuce, there's an excellent chance that the salad is contaminated with bacteria.

To make sure your trip isn't ruined by food poisoning that can cause an upset stomach, diarrhea, nausea, or worse, always travel with probiotics. To boost your first line of defense, two weeks before your departure, take the recommended levels of the "big three" probiotics (L. acidophilus, B. bifidum, and L. bulgaricus), either in capsule or powder form. You need all three of the friendly bacteria to make sure your defensive capabilities are equal to whatever threats may arise.

While you are on your vacation, take your probiotics daily to keep your friendly bacterial forces up to strength. You might want to carry a pocketful of wafers made from L. bulgaricus LB-51 to nibble on at the first sign of stomach upset or indigestion.

If you suffer any signs of food poisoning, I hope you're carrying your powdered probiotics. Remember, food poisoning affects the stomach before it attacks your intestines. Slowly sipping diluted probiotics through a straw will help keep your stomach from rejecting the treatment.

When I travel, I may stay in a small village motel one night, a four-star hotel the next, and an ancient traveler's inn the night after that. Wherever I go, my probiotics go with me, and I see to it that my traveling companions are supplied as well. It pleases me to be able to tell you that I have never had a trip ruined by inadvertently eating spoiled food or drinking bad water. Although I insist that we all avoid as many problems as possible by following the simple rules I outlined above, I rely heavily on a stepped-up intake of friendly bacteria. I know the "home guard" keeps us well protected.

Gastroenteritis.

See Food Poisoning.

Headache.

You can develop a headache at any time of the day or night, while at home, at work, or at play. You can go to bed with a headache or wake up with one. Just about everyone has experienced this common ailment at one time or another.

Headaches can be mild or severe, and occasional or frequent. Although the most common causes of most headaches are stress and tension, other common triggers include eyestrain, sinus problems, head trauma, hormone imbalance, and temperomandibular jaw (TMJ) syndrome. Using certain drugs (including alcohol and tobacco), breathing in polluted air or irritants from perfumes and colognes, and having toxins present in your bloodstream are other likely causes. Conjunctivitis, sinusitis, middle-ear infections, fever, shock, and excitement can all bring on a headache, as well as gastrointestinal disturbances, including constipation, hyper- or hypoacidity, and dyspepsia (a consequence of inadequate digestion).

Probiotics to the rescue. As you will see, many headaches that are caused by the presence of toxins in the bloodstream and / or digestive problems, can be alleviated with the help of your friendly bacteria.

Some forms of headaches are diet-related. Certain foods, including cheese, chocolate, and even wine, can trigger a headache in certain sensitive individuals. This is due to the unfriendly *Streptococcus faecalis* bacteria, which lives alongside the "good guys" in your gastrointestinal tract. *S. faecalis* is one of the normal inhabitants of the human bowel, however, it is also an agent in many urinary tract infections and in subacute endocarditis (an inflammation of the heart). Additionally, it plays a part in causing headaches in certain individuals. You see, *S. faecalis* alters the amino acid tyrosine (a component of many protein foods), and converts it into tyramine, which is a common cause of headaches including migraines. Large quantities of tyramine are typically found in some cheeses, chocolate, and many wines. If you generally come down with a headache after indulging in these foods, it's because you have a sensitivity to this particular protein.

Even those who can enjoy these foods without getting headaches are not "home free" without the services of the friendly bacteria. As I explained earlier in Chapter 2, incompletely digested proteins are one consequence of a friendly bacteria deficiency. When toxins and partially digested proteins are able to permeate the intestinal wall and enter the bloodstream, the immune system will respond by attacking these substances, and headaches are a common result.

In addition, headaches are often one of the common symptoms of a chronic infection. If you suffer from an on-again, off-again infection of the sinuses, nose, middle ear, mouth, or other areas of your body, you are absorbing toxins at a terrific rate. It is not just the stuffed-up sinus cavities that cause pain, it's the absorption of the toxins caused by the bacterial infection that brings on a headache. As stated earlier, friendly bacteria minimize the growth of toxin-producing bacteria. Thus, fewer toxins produce fewer symptoms.

The migraine headache is a vascular headache involving the excessive constriction or dilation of the brain's blood vessels. Although your doctor can't explain why migraines occur, one of the tell-tale symptoms is a disturbance of the gastrointestinal tract. And most of these disturbances can be controlled by adding probiotics to your daily supplement program.

Because some headaches, including migraines, are diet-related, the use of probiotic products that restore a healthy balance to intestinal flora are especially useful. In her 1986 article, "The Shift to Probiotics," published in the *Journal of Alternative Medicine*, Monica Bryant of the University of Sussex reports on her study, which showed that the use of probiotics had "consistently good results with headaches and migraines that are diet-related."

Let me further explain. As discussed above, the *S. faecalis* bacteria can convert the amino acid tyrosine into tyramine, which has been identified as a causative factor in migraine headaches. As explained earlier, tyramine is present in chocolate, some wines, and some cheeses in relatively large quantities. It is known to trigger migraine attacks in sensitive individuals. When the population of friendly bacteria in the bowel falls, leaving the field open to an overgrowth of *S.*

faecalis, tyramine conversion is stepped up. Those individuals who are susceptible to its effects may end up with a blinding migraine. This is why keeping the friendly bacterial guardians of the bowel up to strength can ward off a headache.

RECOMMENDED PROBIOTIC REGIMEN

- When experiencing a headache, take 2 capsules each of *L. acidophilus* and *B. bifidum* (or 1 teaspoon each powder), along with ½ teaspoon *L. bulgaricus* powder mixed in 6 to 8 ounces unchilled filtered water, three times daily before meals.

- Instead of the above regimen, take 1 combination capsule that contain all three super strains in an oil-matrix carrier, three times daily.

- Maintain either of the above regimens as needed for symptomatic relief of headaches. If, after a decrease in either regimen, the headache returns, begin taking the recommended amount again. (Maintenance will depend on how frequently the symptoms return.)

NOTE: For choosing the highest quality probiotics, see guidelines beginning on page 137.

Hyperthyroidism.

Hyperthyroidism develops when the thyroid gland is overactive and produces too much hormone. This condition speeds up the body's processes resulting in symptoms that include rapid and irregular heartbeat, high blood pressure, hands that tremor slightly, constant hunger yet weight loss, fatigue yet increased activity level, heat intolerance, stomach and intestinal spasms, and frequent bowel movements often accompanied by diarrhea. Hyperthyroidism can affect the eyes, including puffiness, irritation, increased tearing, and light sensitivity. Medical treatment includes antithyroid drugs, but surgical removal of the thyroid is sometimes necessary. Left untreated, hyperthyroidism can lead to death due to heart failure.

The most serious form of this condition is Grave's disease. You may remember that both former President George Bush and First Lady Barbara Bush were treated for Grave's disease while he was in office.

Symptoms include those of hyperthyroidism plus a few additional signs, including enlargement of the thyroid gland that results in a bulging neck (goiter), and bulging eyes (exophthalmos).

Yersinia enterocolitica are the harmful intestinal bacteria that are involved with a hyperthyroid condition. This bacteria has the ability to provoke the production of certain substances that attach themselves to cells in the thyroid, resulting in the overproduction of thyroid hormone. More than 80 percent of those with Grave's disease carry antibodies produced by the immune system to destroy *Yersinia*.

Yersinia enterocolitica overgrowth results when these colonies are not kept in check by *L. acidophilus*, *B. bifidum*, and *L. bulgaricus* through competitive exclusion. Once the overgrowth is prevalent, translocation of the bacteria—often through the bloodstream— can occur, making the *Y. enterocolitica* bacteria even more difficult to contain. The importance, therefore, of beneficial bacteria in inhibiting *Y. enterocolitica* is obvious.

RECOMMENDED PROBIOTIC REGIMEN

- Take 2 capsules each of *L. acidophilus* and *B. bifidum* (or 1 teaspoon each powder), along with ½ teaspoon *L. bulgaricus* mixed in 6 to 8 ounces unchilled filtered water, three times daily before meals.

- Instead of the above regimen, take 1 combination capsule that contains all three super strains in an oil-matrix carrier, three times daily.)

NOTE: For choosing the highest quality probiotics, see guidelines beginning on page 137.

Intestinal Neurosis.

See Irritable Bowel Syndrome.

Irritable Bowel Syndrome.

Irritable bowel syndrome (IBS), also referred to as spastic colon, intestinal neurosis, and mucous colitis, is characterized by abnormal muscle contractions of the small and large intestines. It is estimated that one in every five Americans and three times as many women than men suffer from IBS.

In this condition, the gastrointestinal tract is sensitive to many stimuli including stress, diet, and drugs. This sensitivity results in irregular muscle contractions that interfere with the normal transit of food and waste matter. The food and fecal matter pass through the intestines quickly, generally leading to diarrhea. The strong contractions result in cramps (often severe) in the lower abdominal region.

For a true diagnosis of irritable bowel syndrome, your doctor will first want to rule out dysentery and certain inflammatory bowel diseases, such as Crohn's disease. Medical treatment for an irritable bowel usually includes antidiarrheal drugs to reduce the frequency of bowel movements, and bulk-producing agents to give better form to the stool.

The medical profession calls irritable bowel syndrome a "functional disease"—a condition that produces the symptoms of a physical disease, but that reveals no signs of a physical problem upon examination. This doesn't mean that those who suffer from this condition don't have real symptoms or suffer real pain. They do.

When attempting to treat IBS, know that mental as well as physical causes are possible. Anxiety, depression, and emotional stress can trigger the symptoms characteristic of irritable bowel syndrome. But any condition—mental or physical—that affects the gastrointestinal tract can be helped by friendly bacterial supplementation.

The friendly bacteria lactobacilli release essential amino acids during fermentation. Fermented dairy products are rich in several essential amino acids, including tryptophan, which your body uses to produce serotonin—a neurotransmitter with a calming effect. If you've ever had a cup of warm milk at night to help you relax and sleep, know that it is the tryptophan in milk that makes this natural insomnia remedy work. When a cultured milk product, such as real yogurt, is eaten, the action of the friendly bacteria results in even more tryptophan, which, in turn, means more relaxing serotonin. Because the bacteria are so densely concentrated in quality probiotics, taking bacterial supplements may be very effective in helping reduce the stress that can trigger bouts with IBS.

Lactose intolerance (the inability to digest lactose—milk sugar) is another common physical trigger for irritable bowel syndrome. Those who are lactose intolerant are missing the enzyme lactase, which is necessary for the digestion of lactose. Among a number of other beneficial products, the friendly lactobacilli produce lactase to help digest milk and milk products. If your irritable bowel is caused by lactose intolerance, there's an excellent chance that you can overcome the problem through the use of probiotics.

RECOMMENDED PROBIOTIC REGIMEN

- Start with 1 capsule each of *L. acidophilus* and *B. bifidum* (or ½ teaspoon each powder), along with ½ teaspoon *L. bulgaricus* powder mixed in 6 to 8 ounces unchilled filtered water, three times daily before meals.

- Can increase the amount to 3 capsules each of *L. acidophilus* and *B. bifidum* (or 1½ teaspoons each powder), along with 1 tablespoon *L. bulgaricus* powder mixed in 6 to 8 ounces unchilled filtered water, three times daily before meals.

- Instead of the above regimen, can start with 1 combination capsule that contains all three super strains in an oil-matrix carrier, two times daily. Can increase to 1 capsule, four times daily.

Note: For choosing the highest quality probiotics, see guidelines beginning on page 137.

Lactose Intolerance.

Lactose intolerance is the body's inability to digest lactose—a sugar found in milk. Those with this condition are missing the enzyme lactase, which is needed to break down lactose into simple sugars that the body can use. When a person with this condition drinks milk or consumes a milk product, some or all of the product's lactose remains undigested in the intestinal tract. Here, the undigested lactose ferments and commonly causes bloating, abdominal cramps, and diarrhea. About 75 percent of all adults have some degree of lactose intolerance (only Caucasians with origins in northern Europe are able to digest lactose).

Although lactose intolerance can cause discomfort, it is not a serious health threat and can generally be avoided by staying away from foods that contain lactose—primarily dairy products. Unfortunately, this can result in the need for calcium supplementation. The wise use of probiotics can help those who are lactose intolerant. Friendly lactobacilli bacteria produce lactase to help digest milk and milk products.

Keep in mind, however, some people who are unable to digest casein—a milk protein—will exhibit the same symptoms as those who are lactose intolerant. Unfortunately, symptoms of those who are casein intolerant cannot be alleviated by probiotic supplements (see inset on Casein Intolerance, page 41).

RECOMMENDED PROBIOTIC REGIMEN

It is best to start with dairy-based probiotic products, as they produce the most lactase, which is necessary to help your body digest the lactose in milk and milk products. However, some very highly sensitive people may have a reaction to any milk based-product, so it is best to start with very small amounts of probiotics. If there is no reaction, begin to increase the amounts gradually.

- Start with ⅛ teaspoon each of *L. acidophilus, B. bifidum,* and *L. bulgaricus* powders mixed in 6 to 8 ounces unchilled filtered water, taken once a day before any meal. Gradually increase the amount to ¼ teaspoon of each powder, then to ½ teaspoon. (Many who are lactose intolerant are able to take ½ teaspoon of each powder immediately, while others may need to start with smaller amounts.)

- When you are able to take ½ teaspoon of each powder, test your system to see if it is beginning to tolerate lactose. Start by consuming 4 to 6 ounces plain yogurt, once a day. If your body has no adverse reaction, try the same amount of yogurt twice a day. Next, you might introduce a small amount of aged cheese into your diet. The important thing is to introduce the foods in small amounts and gradually. If you continue to experience symptoms of lactose intolerance, increase the oral regimen presented above, then start testing your system again. Continue testing until symptoms of lactose intolerance subside.

NOTE: For choosing the highest quality probiotics, see guidelines beginning on page 137.

Listeriosis.

See Food Poisoning.

Migraine Headache.

See Headache.

Mouth Sores.

See Canker Sores; Cold Sores.

Mucous Colitis.

See Irritable Bowel Syndrome.

Osteoporosis.

Osteoporosis is a progressive disease resulting in loss of normal bone density. The bones become thin, porous, and brittle, making the individual susceptible to bone fractures. Loss of body height also occurs as the disease progresses. Osteoporosis primarily affects women. The amount of mineral in the bone—bone mass—reaches a peak when a woman is between thirty and thirty-five years old. Typically, as a woman gets older, bone loss occurs.

Insufficient calcium intake is a major factor that causes osteoporosis, but there are other dietary practices that affect calcium metabolism as well. For instance, a high-sugar or high-sodium diet, or a diet high in animal protein, causes the body to excrete increased amounts of needed calcium. This forces the body to get the calcium it needs from bones. Other products that cause these same results include caffeine, alcohol, and a variety of drugs. Regular weight-bearing exercise, like walking, is recommended for increasing bone mass. And calcium and magnesium supplements in a ratio of two to one are often recommended to prevent or slow down the negative effects of osteoporosis.

The disease is also tied to a deficiency of the female hormone estrogen, and is seen most often in postmenopausal women. Declining estrogen production or the inability to assimilate calcium normally disturbs the calcium balance, leading to bone porosity and brittleness. Calcium is normally absorbed by bone. The calcium content of bone is regulated and maintained by estrogen and parathyroid hormones. Without normal estrogen levels, calcium is actually leached out of the bones and ends up being deposited in the soft tissues of the body.

When the normal colonies of beneficial flora in the gastrointestinal tract are depleted for any reason, changes occur that cause excessive amounts of estrogen to be eliminated, instead of being recycled. The end result is that very low levels of this important hormone are present in the bloodstream. Another reason to keep your friendly bacteria levels strong is that they produce lactic acid, which has been shown to have a positive effect on the improved utilization and absorption of calcium.

RECOMMENDED PROBIOTIC REGIMEN

- Take 1 teaspoon each of *L. acidophilus, B. bifidum,* and *L. bulgaricus* powders mixed in 8 ounces plain yogurt, twice daily.
- In addition to the above regimen, for increased strength, take 1 combination capsule that contains all three super strains in an oil-matrix carrier, once a day.

NOTE: For choosing the highest quality probiotics, see guidelines beginning on page 137.

Radiation Sickness.

Exposure to radioactive substances causes radiation sickness. This can be the result of brief exposure to high levels of radiation or long-term exposure to low levels. Ionizing radiation destroys or damages cells, which can lead to cancer. Mutations in the genetic makeup of cells in the sexual organs can result in birth defects in offspring.

Harmful high-level radiation once came from diagnostic x-rays. Fortunately, modern technological diagnostic procedures produce much less radiation than in the past. The most common high-level radiation sources today are man-made radioactive materials that are used in nuclear power plants and in a number of medical procedures. They do not come from x-rays. Acute symptoms of high-level radiation, although relatively uncommon, are dangerous. Generally beginning with nausea and vomiting, listlessness, and general weakness, the symptoms progress to dehydration, convulsions, and even death.

Radiation sickness as the result of low-level radiation exposure commonly has symptoms that include dizziness, headache, fatigue, and nausea. Common low-level exposure sources are medical and dental x-rays, radon or uranium present in building materials, tobacco smoke, cellular phones, computer monitors, satellite dishes, and microwave ovens. Those who work in nuclear power plants, or in an industry that produces radioactive material for medical or industrial purposes, have greater chances of radiation exposure.

Of course, the type and extent of the damage caused by radiation exposure depends on a number of factors—the total dose and length of time of exposure, the area of the body affected, and the size of the area exposed.

During radiation therapy for cancer patients, high doses of radiation are specifically targeted at malignant cells. This treatment kills the cancer with minimal involvement of the surrounding healthy tissue. Radiation sickness is this treatment's major side effect.

In Chapter 9, "The Anti-Cancer Capabilities of Friendly Bacteria," you saw how strong colonies of friendly bacteria can lighten the immune system's workload, keeping it strong in the fight against harmful microorganisms. Studies also show that *L. bulgaricus* super strain LB-51, helps lessen the destructive side effects of chemotherapy and radiation treatment.

The work of Drs. K.M. Shahani, G.V. Reddy, and A.M. Joe shows that the friendly bacteria may be able to ward off birth defects in children whose parents have been exposed to radiation. In their 1974 work entitled, "Nutritional and Therapeutic Aspects of Cultured Dairy Products," they reported on their work with guinea pigs that had been deliberately exposed to radiation. The guinea pigs were divided into two groups. One group was given acidophilus milk daily, while the control group received none. Offspring born to the control group suffered a great number of serious deformities. Litters born to those who received the acidophilus milk were normal; none had birth defects. These offspring developed better and gained more weight than those in the control group. This *in vivo* study was proof of the friendly bacteria's efficacy in preventing birth defects in laboratory animals who had been exposed to radiation.

Similar effects have been observed in humans. In the book *Natural Sources* by researchers Moira Timms and Zacharia Zar, the authors state that the daily consumption of between a pint and a quart of yogurt (or soured milk) has been found to eliminate residues of radioactive strontium 90 from the bowel.

We also know that regular use of cultured milk products improves one's general nutritional status and results in a measurable reduction of toxic elements in the bowel and bloodstream.

RECOMMENDED PROBIOTIC REGIMEN

The following probiotic regimen is recommended for anyone undergoing chemotherapy or radiation therapy, as well as those who work in nuclear power plants or diagnostic laboratories in which x-rays are administered.

- Take ½ teaspoon each of *L. acidophilus*, *B.bifidum*, and *L. bulgaricus* powders mixed together in 6 to 8 ounces unchilled filtered water, or mix the powders in 8 ounces plain yogurt, two to three times daily.
- In addition to or instead of the above regimen, for increased strength, take 1 combination capsule that contains all three super strains in an oil-matrix carrier, one to three times daily.

NOTE: For choosing the highest quality probiotics, see guidelines beginning on page 137.

Rheumatoid Arthritis.

Like Crohn's disease, rheumatoid arthritis (RA) is an autoimmune disease. RA causes the body to attack the synovial membranes, which secrete the lubricating fluid in the joints. This results in joint inflammation and the destruction of connective tissue and cartilage surrounding the joints.

Symptoms include joint stiffness, tenderness, and swelling, as well as fatigue, anemia, and crippling pain. Further, painful arthritic nodes at pressure points, such as the elbows, develop. In the final Stage IV of the disease, the patient generally has joint defects, muscle destruction, soft tissue tumors, and bone and cartilage degeneration, as well as ankylosis—a joining of the joints.

Medical treatment includes rest, exercise to improve joint function, drugs to reduce pain and inflammation, surgery to prevent or correct defects, and a nutritional diet. Steroids are given with caution because of their known side effects.

In the case of rheumatoid arthritis, the tissue type most frequently found in patients is HL-DR4. The bacteria that most closely matches the characteristics of HL-DR4 is *Proteus*, a common cause of urinary tract infections. Interestingly enough, women—who have a much higher rate of urinary tract infections than men—also suffer from rheumatoid arthritis twice as often as men.

Once *Proteus* was identified as close in characteristic to HL-DR4 tissue types, it was a simple matter of testing Dr. Alan Ebringer's theory, which states the body's immune system could make a mistake in its efforts to get rid of an undesirable bacteria, and be fooled into attacking its own tissues instead. When levels of *Proteus* antibodies found in the blood of people with rheumatoid arthritis were compared with those of healthy people, the antibodies were discovered to be much higher.

When strong armies of beneficial bacteria are on guard to control the overgrowth of *Proteus*, many symptoms of rheumatoid arthritis can be eliminated.

RECOMMENDED PROBIOTIC REGIMEN

In addition to the following probiotic regimen, those with rheumatoid arthritis may consider taking 1 tablespoon of emulsified cod liver oil, which helps to minimize pain.

- Take 2 capsules each of *L. acidophilus* and *B. bifidum* (or 1 teaspoon each powder) along with ½ teaspoon *L. bulgaricus* powder mixed in 6 to 8 ounces unchilled filtered water, three times daily.

- In addition to or instead of the above regimen, for increased strength, take 1 combination capsule that contains all three super strains in an oil-matrix carrier, one to three times daily.

NOTE: For choosing the highest quality probiotics, see guidelines beginning on page 137.

Salmonellosis.

See Food Poisoning.

Scalded Skin Syndrome.

Scalded Skin Syndrome (SSS) is a potentially deadly widespread skin infection that typically affects babies, young children, and those with depressed immune systems. It is caused by toxins that are secreted by the insidious *Staphylococcus aureus* bacteria. (For additional information on *S. aureus* bacteria, see the inset on page 208.)

SSS usually spreads from a primary infection such as conjunctivitis. Symptoms include fever, profound weakness, and bright red skin. The skin develops large blisters that slough off in sheets, leaving large areas of the body without skin at all. Even normal-looking skin falls away with the slightest pressure. The loss of skin is terribly serious because it exposes the area to widespread infection. It also upsets the body's temperature controls and fluid-balance mechanisms.

The prompt use of antibiotics is the medical treatment of choice. It is very important to take supplemental friendly bacteria both during and after antibiotic treatment in order to keep the friendly bacteria in strong numbers.(See Probiotic Use During Antibiotic Treatment on page 139.)

RECOMMENDED PROBIOTIC REGIMEN

- Between prescribed doses of antibiotics, take 2 capsules each of *L. acidophilus* and *B. bifidum* (or 1 to 2 teaspoons each powder), along with 1 teaspoon *L. bulgaricus* powder mixed with 6 to 8 ounces unchilled filtered water, three times daily.

- In addition to or instead of the above regimen, for increased strength, take 1 combination capsule that contains all three super strains, three times daily.

- For at least 2 weeks following antibiotic treatment, double or triple the above regimen.

NOTE: For choosing the highest quality probiotics, see guidelines beginning on page 137.

Skin Problems. *See also* Acne.

Your skin does a great deal more than just hold your bones, muscles, and organs in place. It also acts as a barrier against environmental pollutants, contaminants, and harmful bacteria. More than just a protective covering, your skin—actually the largest organ of your body—is able to rid itself of toxins that are not excreted through urine or fecal matter.

Bacterial toxins that exit through your skin can cause allergies, rashes, and serious skin conditions, including eczema, psoriasis, and acne. This is why many dermatologists routinely prescribe powerful oral or topical antibiotics—tetracycline is a favorite—to help minimize the infections caused by bacterial overgrowth. Unfortunately, antibiotics kill the friendly bacteria as well the harmful ones. And you need the help of your friendly bacteria to handle the infectious bacteria that comes from both the inside-out and the outside-in.

Your skin consists of two layers: the outer epidermis and the underlying dermis. The epidermis is a thin, relatively transparent layer that is divided into three layers. Outer dead skin cells are regularly sloughed off as the result of washing, as well as everyday pressure and friction. The sloughed-off cells are replaced by newer skin cells that have been manufactured in the blood-rich base layers of the epidermis. New skin cells naturally rise to the outer surface of your skin over the course of about thirty days. In the natural order of things, these cells gradually die as they become increasingly thinner and flatter.

Under ideal circumstances, your skin is a naturally replenishing organ. The trouble, of course, is that "ideal" circumstances seldom exist. You are constantly being bombarded by "bad" bacteria, both from the outside and the inside. Young facial skin is prone to acne and blemishes, but the problems change as we get older. As the body ages, the natural replenishing process becomes less efficient and the skin becomes drier, less elastic. Just as young skin is fertile ground for pimples, older and drier skin is prone to creases and wrinkles. After menopause, especially, the outer layer of skin cells take much longer to renew. The cumulative effects of exposure to the sun can cause the skin to become thick and leathery. And smoking ages skin faster than almost any other factor.

Over the last few years, alpha-hydroxy acids have been touted as

Probiotics for Your Skin

A proprietary probiotic face cream formula that employs modern science and cutting-age technology to update the secrets of ancient beauties is now available in most health food stores. This product began with an analysis of the specific beneficial components inherent in cultured milk products. These components include DNA fragments of beneficial bacterial cells, natural proteolytic enzymes that are helpful and specific for the face, and natural antimicrobial substances that can eliminate nasty bacteria that may infect the skin from both the outside and the inside. Because they enhance the natural process the skin uses to repair itself, the DNA fragments alone are the most important active ingredients in the cream.

These components are dispersed in a special oxygenated aloe vera base that actually affects the skin at its molecular level where new cells are born. Although aloe vera is thought to be very soothing, you might be surprised to learn that it carries a possible irritant. If you've ever cut a piece of aloe vera, you know that the bright green interior quickly turns a brownish-yellow. This color change is the result of a compound called sinoil, which carries irritants. The probiotic cream, however, uses a very pure, enzyme-activated, sinoil-free form of aloe vera as its base, thus allowing all the important components of the formula to permeate the epidermis without irritation. Because surface cells "communicate" with lower-level cells, the benefits reach down deep into the dermis.

Observation has shown that the probiotic cream gently speeds up the natural exfoliation process and helps oxygenate the skin at the molecular level. The result is similar to that of alpha-hydroxy acids, only without the redness, irritation, and skin damage that often results. With probiotic cream, many women have experienced almost instantaneous soothing and calming effects on areas of facial skin that had been severely irritated by products containing alpha-hydroxy acids.

While ridding the skin of dead surface cells, probiotic cream—thanks to the important DNA components—is extremely gentle and will not harm the underlying layers. The special bacterial factors help normalize the complex biochemistry of the skin, minimizing the activity of harmful bacteria that are potentially infectious. Probiotic cream preserves and promotes the natural acid mantle of the skin—one of nature's defenses against harmful environmental pollutants. It also aids in the reduction of pore size.

With regular use, probiotic cream reinforces those natural processes that keep the skin young and fresh. It normalizes oil production, but promotes moisture retention, resulting in skin that has a youthful glow without being greasy. The cream's enzymes gently accelerate the natural exfoliation process of the skin while diminishing fine lines and wrinkles. Minimizing the signs of aging, this cream actually "youthproofs" the skin by firming, toning, and tightening it—effects you can feel the first time and every time you use it. Recommended by leading dermatologists, this cream, which benefits all skin types, is the only one necessary. However, it can be used in conjunction with other creams, lotions, or sunscreens, if you wish.

Probiotic cream leaves your face soft and smooth and ready for makeup, if desired. After using the cream regularly, many women say that they don't bother with makeup anymore because the appearance of their "naked" skin has become so pleasing. It not only insures clean, clear, smooth skin, it's also the best way to retain skin's youthful properties.

For optimal results, while using this skin cream, be sure to take the "big three" probiotics (L. acidophilus, B. bifidum, and L. bulgaricus) in powder or capsule form daily. Just like all the other systems of your body, healthy skin begins within.

Presently, a probiotic formula for a facial mask is being "field tested" by selected subjects. When perfected, this mask may eliminate the need for certain types of plastic surgery, including chemical peels and laser "lifts." Keep an eye out for this product.

super facial skin-exfoliators—they speed up the natural sloughing off process. Therein, however, lies the problem. Often, the dead cells are removed too quickly, uncovering new cells that are too young to be exposed to the air. The result is reddened, irritated skin.

Through the legendary beauties of ancient civilizations, we have learned that cultured milk was used both as food and beauty treatment. It is written that Cleopatra bathed in the fermented milk of asses. We also know that women from areas where cultured dairy products are a staple are noted for the exceptional clarity and beauty of their skin. A probiotic skin cream is now available that can eliminate harmful bacteria that may harm the skin. (See Probiotics for Your Skin, beginning on page 202.)

Young or old, male or female, everyone wants clean, clear, smooth skin. Glowing skin is an excellent sign of good health, both inside and out.

RECOMMENDED PROBIOTIC REGIMEN

- Take 1 capsule each of *L. acidophilus* and *B. bifidum* (or ½ teaspoon each powder), along with ½ teaspoon *L. bulgaricus* powder mixed in 6 to 8 ounces unchilled filtered water, three times daily.
- Instead of the above regimen, take 1 combination capsule that contains all three super strains in an oil-matrix carrier, once daily.
- Apply probiotic skin cream (see inset on page 202) to your face and neck each morning and evening for healthy skin.
- For skin with acne or an occasional outbreak of pimples, stronger topical action may be desired. See Acne entry for directions on how to make a probiotic paste for the skin.

NOTE: For choosing the highest quality probiotics, see guidelines beginning on page 137.

Spastic Colon.

See Irritable Bowel Syndrome.

Staphylococcus aureus Poisoning.

See Food Poisoning.

Stress.

See also Anxiety; Depression.

Any physical, mental, or emotional stimulus that upsets the natural balance of the body is referred to as stress. We encounter stressful situations on a daily basis. Some causes are obvious, such as the breakup of an important relationship, illness of a loved one, pressures at work, or mounting bills. Other, less obvious stressors may come from sitting in traffic, waiting in long lines at the bank or grocery store, or being stuck in the middle of a crowded or noisy environment. Anxiety over upcoming events, such as the birth of a new baby, the start of a new job, or an impending speech can cause stress.

Emotional stress, which can result in fatigue, headache, insomnia, high blood pressure, irritability, and gastrointestinal disorders, can lead to other, more serious illnesses, such as cardiovascular disease, cancer, back problems, and infections. Stress is also a possible cause of depression. Stress typically affects those parts of the body related to the nervous system—especially the gastrointestinal tract.

Stress causes an increase in adrenaline, which triggers a release of stored sugar (energy) from your liver. In response to this rush of adrenaline, blood is diverted from your intestines to your muscles, which causes a dramatic slowdown of your digestive processes. Chronic stress causes a constant digestive slowdown, which compromises the health of your friendly bacteria.

If this pattern continues over a long period of time, the most obvious effects occur in the large intestine. The colon can suffer actual damage to its inner surface lining. Swelling, inflammation, and even some localized miniature hemorrhages can occur. Depending on which bacteria are present in the damaged region and which dietary substances are passing through, a variety of toxic substances can build up. Some of these toxins can migrate through the damaged intestinal lining into your bloodstream, with serious consequences.

Anyone with chronic bowel dysfunction should make every effort to cut down on the stress in their lives, or, better yet, try to modify their reaction to it. Stress-reducing methods that work include breathing and relaxation techniques, meditation, and visualization.

In sufficient strength, the friendly lactobacteria can indirectly help in alleviating stress. During fermentation, lactobacilli release essential amino acids, including tryptophan. Tryptophan produces seratonin— a calming neurotransmitter. Tryptophan is found in milk, which is why drinking a glass of warm milk is a traditional cure for insomnia. Cultured milk products like real yogurt, contain even more tryptophan, and high-quality lactobacteria supplements contain the most.

While there is no hard evidence that lactobacilli directly alleviates stress, its release of tryptophan may indirectly help to encourage a relaxing, calming state. Taking supplemental lactobacteria appears to be a step in the right direction.

RECOMMENDED PROBIOTIC REGIMEN

- Take 1 capsule each of *L. acidophilus* and *B. bifidum* (or ½ teaspoon powder), along with ½ teaspoon *L. bulgaricus* powder mixed in 6 to 8 ounces unchilled filtered water, two times daily. May be increased to 2 capsules *L acidophilus* and *B. bifidum* (or 1 teaspoon powder), and 1 teaspoon *L. bulgaricus* powder, three times daily.

- Instead of the above regimen, take 1 or 2 combination capsules that contain all three super strains in an oil-matrix carrier, once a day.

- For times when under stress, and experiencing "butterflies" (or worse) in your stomach, mix ½ teaspoon each of *L. acidophilus*, *B. bifidum*, and *L. bulgaricus* powders together in 6 to 8 ounces unchilled filtered water, and sip it slowly through a straw. This will have a calming effect.

NOTE: For choosing the highest quality probiotics, see guidelines beginning on page 137.

Toxic Bowel. *See also* Ankylosing Spondylitis; Crohn's Disease; Hyperthyroidism; Rheumatoid Arthritis; and Ulcerative Colitis.

Highly toxic substances are produced in your intestinal tract. Your friendly bacteria protect you against most of these toxins, as long as sufficient numbers are on duty. However, when the friendly bacteria are caught off guard, you can end up with what is known as a "toxic bowel." This can lead to a serious problem called autotoxemia, or self-poisoning. A dysfunctional intestinal tract is the direct result of a deficiency of the friendly bacteria.

As pathogens spread and overgrow, they can eventually take a "bite" out of the intestinal wall, causing microinfections. This also allows the toxins to permeate the wall and get into the bloodstream and nervous system. The immune system must jump into the act at this point and try to rid the body of these toxins. The result? A weakened immune system.

There are some serious medical conditions that can be tied to toxic bowel problems. Autoimmune diseases that are known to have a toxic bowel connection include ankylosing spondylitis, Crohn's disease, hyperthyroidism, rheumatoid arthritis, and ulcerative colitis. Other conditions such as toxic shock syndrome (TSS) and scalded skin syndrome (SSS) are the direct result of the proliferation of one of the most damaging bacterias of all—*Staphylococcus aureus* (see inset on page 208).

To prevent a buildup of toxins in the intestinal tract, it is very important to keep your friendly bacteria strong. If, however, you are already suffering with a toxic bowel, it is important to begin a probiotic regimen.

RECOMMENDED PROBIOTIC REGIMEN

When beginning a probiotic regimen to combat a toxic bowel, it is important to realize that, depending on the level of toxicity, the die-off of toxins may result in the Herxheimer Reaction—gas, bloating, and possible headaches (see inset on page 148). Depending on the discomfort level you are willing to handle, it may be best to start by taking minimal amounts of probiotics, gradually increasing their amount and frequency as you see fit.

- Start with 1 capsule each of *L. acidophilus* and *B. bifidum* (or ½ teaspoon each powder), along with ½ teaspoon *L. bulgaricus* powder, mixed in 6 to 8 ounces unchilled filtered water, three times daily.

- Gradually increase the *L. acidophilus* and *B. bifidum* to 3 capsules (or 1 to 2 teaspoons powder), and the *L. bulgaricus* powder to 2 teaspoons.

NOTE: For choosing the highest quality probiotics, see guidelines beginning on page 137.

The Harmful Effects of Staphylococcus aureus

Staphylococcus aureus is a particularly nasty organism that lives in the mucous membranes that line the nose, mouth, intestinal tract, and vagina. In its mildest form, it can cause boils, carbuncles, and internal abscesses. Other conditions associated with S. aureus include gastroenteritis, bone and joint infections (osteomyelitis), septic arthritis, toxic shock syndrome (TSS), scalded skin syndrome (SSS), pneumonia, meningitis, and inflammatory heart disease (endocarditis). When the friendly bacteria that keep S. aureus bacteria under control are depleted, this harmful bacteria is allowed to proliferate and wreak havoc.

Food contaminated with the toxins produced by S. aureus account for 25 percent of all food poisoning cases. The contamination typically occurs when a food handler with a staphylococcal skin infection touches food that is left to sit out at room temperature. This enables the bacteria to proliferate and produce toxins. As the staphylococci microorganism is typically found in the nose and throat, food can also become contaminated if it is sneezed or coughed on.

In all bacterial infections, the first line of defense is the use of a broad-spectrum antibiotic. Unfortunately, hospital studies show that around 90 percent of S. aureus infections have become resistant to most known antibiotics. In addition, the troublemaking Candida albicans yeast-fungus, actually helps S. aureus do its work. In her 1983 paper, "Enhancement by Candida of S. aureus, Serratia marcescens, and S. faecalis in the Establishment of Infection," published in Infection and Immunity, Dr. Eunice Carlson demonstrated that when there is a combined infection of S. aureus (or S. faecalis or Serratia marcescens) accompanied by candida overgrowth, there is an increase in the strength of the bacteria.

Dr. Carlson states, "Although these studies show that candida has a strong amplifying effect on the virulence of other organisms, how this is achieved is a mystery. One possibility is that the candidal infection process causes physical damage to the organ walls, which makes them 'leaky,' allowing other microbes or chemicals (perhaps toxins) or both to penetrate more easily; it is also possible that candida directly stimulates the growth of S. aureus."

> One reason many doctors fail to either identify or treat candida aggressively is because they either don't recognize that it is part of the problem, or they cannot prove its presence. Dr. Carlson refers to the known infestation of dentures with candida, saying, "It is now believed to be very common and to occur in 60 percent of all denture wearers. Biopsies of inflamed areas, however, consistently fail to demonstrate tissue invasion [by candida]. We can speculate that an equivalent infection of the small intestine would be virtually undetectable."
>
> Dr. Carlson continues, "Physicians have reported therapeutic cures for a variety of diverse disease conditions by anticandidal drugs. It now appears possible that this fungus may play a key role in many disease conditions, not by its own toxic or invasive growth, but rather by enhancing secondary infection."
>
> We know that strong colonies of friendly bacteria are well able to handle both candida and staph infections. Many doctors are becoming aware that the best approach to correcting the toxic bowel or any bacterial involvement of the gastrointestinal tract is by supplementing with friendly bacteria.

Toxic Liver.

A very wide range of the toxic substances produced in a toxic bowel is sent on to the liver, which is the body's primary detoxification site. A healthy liver neutralizes these toxins, then either recycles them for use in the body, or excretes them. However, an unhealthy liver—one that has been compromised due to illness, improper diet, or drug and/or alcohol abuse, for example, cannot effectively process harmful toxins. Take ammonia, for example.

During the digestion of proteins, a number of harmful bacteria, including *Clostridia*, *Eubacteria*, and *Peptostreptococci*, produce toxic ammonia in the gastrointestinal tract. It is the result of a perfectly normal process. A healthy liver detoxifies the ammonia by turning it into urea, which is passed out of the body in the urine. However, if your liver is not working properly, the ammonia remains unprocessed and can enter the bloodstream and invade the central nervous system, causing many dangerous symptoms. Even your brain can be affected. In advanced cases of cirrhosis of the liver, for example, a mild mental aberration may progress to coma and, ultimately, death. Increased levels of ammonia in the blood are characteristic of liver failure.

Medical treatment of liver disease generally begins by limiting the amount of dietary protein, which adds to ammonia production. The amino acids found in meat produce more ammonia during breakdown than the proteins in milk. Bowel cleansing through the use of laxatives, purgatives, enemas, and colonic irrigation is recommended to remove any putrefying residue.

While antibiotics are routinely prescribed to kill ammonia-producing bacteria for a toxic bowel and toxic liver, unfortunately, they will also kill off many of the friendly bacteria. This depletion of friendly bacteria inevitably will leave the field wide open to even more problems in the gastrointestinal tract, such as the proliferation of the aggressive *C. candida* yeast microorganism. Fortunately, probiotics provide a better alternative.

In their 1983 book, *Bifidobacteria and Their Role*, Drs. J.L. Rasic and J.A. Kurmann explain the use of a bifidogenic diet. This type of diet includes foods and substances that support the action of bifidobacteria in the gastrointestinal tract. One such substance is lactulose, which is helpful in treating patients with advanced liver disease by preventing the absorption of ammonia from the colon.

When lactulose reaches the intestines, it is welcomed by the friendly bacteria as a good food source. Through fermentation, the bacteria turn lactulose into lactic and acetic acids, which help increase the size of the bacterial colonies. This has the natural effect of reducing the pH level of the large intestine, making it far more acidic. When a high level of acidity is present, the ammonia remains in its ionized form. In this form, it is not passed on to the liver or diffused into general circulation through the blood. This reduces the toxic load on the liver and reduces ammonia levels throughout the body, including the brain.

Lactulose not only helps reestablish healthy bowel flora by increasing their numbers, it also helps in reducing the territories of undesirable *Enterobacteria*, *Clostridia*, and *Staphylococci*. One study reported by Dr. Rasic involved twelve patients with cirrhosis of the liver. The average level of the subjects' friendly bacteria was approximately 1 million per gram of feces, while the potentially harmful *E. coli* were highly active at a population level of 100 billion per gram. After these patients had been given lactulose, levels of lactobacteria rose to between 10 and 100 million per gram while the *E. coli* populations decreased dramatically.

To help bring an overloaded, dysfunctional liver back to normal, in addition to lactulose, Dr. Rasic also suggests adding new colonies of bifidobacteria through direct supplementation. One study described by Drs. Rasic and Kurmann, involved thirty-three patients with various degrees of cirrhosis of the liver. At the start of the study, the patients were given 10 grams of a reconstituted bifidus milk product that contained live bifidobacteria three times daily for three years. The dose was gradually increased to 100 grams, three times daily. The study showed a general improvement in the health of these patients, which was confirmed by a decrease in ammonia and free phenol levels, an increase in acidity, and a dramatic increase in bifidobacteria.

In 1968, Dr. D. Muting and colleagues reported their research on the subject of friendly bacteria and the liver in a paper entitled, "The Effect of Bacterium Bifidum on Intestinal Bacterial Flora and Toxic Protein Metabolites in Chronic Liver Disease," published in the *American Journal of Protology*. The researchers conducted a trial involving twenty patients suffering from serious liver disease. These patients, who had no dietary restrictions, were given bifidus milk each day. Within seven to ten days, levels of blood ammonia, serum phenol, and other toxins dropped to normal levels.

Dr. Muting points out the advantages of using bifidus milk over lactulose due to their respective protein levels. Lactulose is a carbohydrate derived from milk sugar, but bifidus milk offers around 30 to 40 percent protein, which is a distinct advantage, especially for severely ill patients.

Although it has been shown that large and healthy colonies of bifidobacteria have the ability to flush harmful ammonia, phenols, and amines from the intestinal tract very quickly, I am not suggesting that serious liver dysfunction is something you can or should treat yourself. More and more health care professionals are becoming aware that direct supplementation of viable friendly bacteria is indicated when the liver and/or gastrointestinal tract are impaired. Discuss this need with your doctor.

When choosing a *Bifidobacterium bifidum* supplement, be sure that the product comes from a dairy-based formula that contains billions of microorganisms per gram and also retains the bacteria's important growing medium—the supernatant. It is this supernatant that contains large amounts of lactulose. Be sure the watchwords "supernatant" and "dairy-based" appear on the label to be assured of a quality product. (For additional information on the supernatant, see inset on page 115.)

Your first priority in self-care health care is tending to the friendly bacteria in your gastrointestinal tract. Not only do they protect you against the serious consequences of a toxic bowel, they also prevent the kind of secondary involvement that leads to the development of a toxic liver.

RECOMMENDED PROBIOTIC REGIMEN

For this particular condition, dairy-based probiotic powders are preferred.

- Take 1 capsule *L. acidophilus* (or ½ teaspoon powder), plus 3 *B. bifidum* capsules (or 2 teaspoons powder), and ½ teaspoon *L. bulgaricus* powder mixed in 6 to 8 ounces unchilled filtered water, three times daily.

- Instead of the above regimen, take 2 combination capsules that contain all three super strains in an oil-matrix carrier, two to three times daily.

NOTE: For choosing the highest quality probiotics, see guidelines beginning on page 137.

Toxic Shock Syndrome.

Usually caused by a monstrous infestation of the *Staphylococcus aureus* bacteria, toxic shock syndrome (TSS), although uncommon, appears mainly in young menstruating women who use tampons. *S. aureus* is a particularly nasty organism that lives in the body's mucous membranes, including those of the nose, mouth, intestinal tract, and vagina. (For more information on harmful *S. aureus* bacteria, see page 208.)

Symptoms of TSS generally begin with a sudden high fever (usually 102°F or higher) that is quickly followed by intense headache, sore throat, fatigue, vomiting, diarrhea, dizziness, muscle aches, lightheadedness, and a rash that looks like a sunburn.

TSS came to public attention in the 1980s when 700 cases were reported. Although the cause is unknown, indications suggest that the presence of a tampon may encourage the *S. aureus* bacteria to produce a toxin that permeates the vaginal lining and enters the bloodstream.

Prompt diagnosis and aggressive treatment with antibiotics are critical. To reduce the risk of TSS, use feminine napkins instead of tampons. If you continue to use tampons, however, alternate them with feminine napkins, and be sure to change them frequently. The majority of reported cases occur in those using super absorbancy products.

Interestingly, each of the reported patients who were diagnosed with TSS, also had a vaginal yeast infection. The presence of yeast encourages the staphylococcus bacteria to grow 500 percent faster than when it is not present.

Healthy vaginal flora is a key to minimizing the consequences of disease-causing bacteria. The daily supplementation of proper probiotics is, therefore, a prudent strategy.

RECOMMENDED PROBIOTIC REGIMEN

- Take 1 capsule each of *L. acidophilus* and *B. bifidum* (or ½ teaspoon each powder), and ½ teaspoon *L. bulgaricus* powder mixed in 6 to 8 ounces unchilled filtered water, two times daily.
- Can increase to 3 capsules each *L. acidophilus* and *B. bifidum* (or 2 teaspoons each powder), and 2 teaspoons *L. bulgaricus* powder, three times daily.
- Instead of the above regimen, take 1 combination capsule that contains all three super strains in an oil-matrix carrier, one to three times daily.

NOTE: For choosing the highest quality probiotics, see guidelines beginning on page 137.

Ulcerative Colitis.

Ulcerative colitis is a chronic disease in which the mucous membranes lining the large intestine become inflamed and ulcerated. This results in fever, abdominal cramps, and bloody diarrhea. Ulcerative colitis usually doesn't affect the entire thickness of the intestine (like Crohn's disease) and never affects the small intestine. This disease usually begins in the rectum or lower end of the large intestine. Unchecked, it can eventually spread partially or completely through the large intestine.

Ulcerative colitis can range from fairly mild to severe. Severe attacks can come on suddenly, producing high fever, violent attacks of diarrhea, and intense abdominal cramps. Other episodes may come on gradually with symptoms of mild lower abdominal cramps, accompanied by stool that contains blood and mucus. The farther up the intestine this disease extends, the more severe the symptoms.

Although the cause of ulcerative colitis is not known, contributing factors may include stress, poor diet, food allergies, heredity, and overactive immune system responses in the intestine. Colitis may also be the result of harmful bacterial overgrowth, often caused by the use of antibiotics.

The link between bacterial overgrowth and certain autoimmune diseases has been confirmed in research centers around the globe. Research is ongoing to identify particular bowel bacteria that may have similar characteristics to tissue types that are commonly found in people with other autoimmune diseases, such as myasthenia gravis, lupus erythematosus, motor neuron disease, and pernicious anemia.

In order to control the inflammation and other symptoms of ulcerative colitis, treatment usually centers around diet. Raw fruits and vegetables as well as dairy products should be avoided. Supplemental high-quality probiotics is recommended to help strengthen the intestinal walls with friendly bacteria.

RECOMMENDED PROBIOTIC REGIMEN

- Start with 1 capsule each *L. acidophilus* and *B. bifidum* (or ½ teaspoon each powder), along with ½ teaspoon *L. bulgaricus* powder mixed in 6 to 8 ounces unchilled filtered water, three times daily before meals.

- Can increase the above amount to 3 capsules each of *L. acidophilus* and *B. bifidum* (or 1½ teaspoons powder), and 1 tablespoon *L. bulgaricus* powder, three times daily before meals.

- Instead of the above regimens, can take 1 combination capsule that contains all three super strains in an oil-matrix carrier, two times daily, and increase to 1 capsule, three to four times daily.

NOTE: For choosing the highest quality probiotics, see guidelines beginning on page 137.

Urinary Tract Infection.

The urogenital tract (vagina, cervix, periurethra, and urethra) is a haven for many bacterial species. The bacterial ecology in this area is dynamic and subject to easy change. Therefore, maintaining an optimal balance of the beneficial flora is very important.

Many factors, such as recurring vaginal infections (80 percent of all women) or urinary tract infections (20 percent of all women), can upset the delicate flora balance in the urogenital tract.

Symptoms of urinary tract infection (UTI) include strong or foul-smelling urine, fever, vomiting, diarrhea, irritability, and pain while urinating. The conventional treatment for UTI is antibiotics. Unfortunately, the infection usually recurs once the antibiotic regimen has ended. In some cases, antibiotic-resistant disease-causing bacteria develop and proliferate, producing toxic side effects (see Probiotic Use During Antibiotic Treatment, page 139). In some cases, UTIs are related to vaginal yeast overgrowth. In such cases, the use of antibiotics are ineffective and may actually provoke the yeast to proliferate more vigorously, and encourage the infection to return with added pain and discomfort.

In women, the urethra is short and the opening is very close to the anus, making it prone to contamination from fecal bacteria. Good hygiene in this area, therefore, is highly recommended. After urinating or moving your bowels, always wipe from front to back. In addition, take daily showers and wash vaginal and rectal areas carefully. Avoid bubble baths, and choose to wear "breathable" cotton underwear.

Most important, maintain a daily probiotic supplement program that includes *L. acidophilus*, *B. bifidum*, and *L. bulgaricus* super strains. Balancing the urogenital and gastrointestinal flora to optimize the presence of *L. acidophilus* will play a long-lasting role in preventing vaginal and urinary tract infections. For more detailed information on the positive effects of probiotics on urinary tract infections, see discussion beginning on page 82 in Chapter 7, "The Antibiotic Action of Friendly Bacteria."

RECOMMENDED PROBIOTIC REGIMEN

- If you are diagnosed with a urinary tract infection, take 2 capsules each of *L. acidolphilus* and *B. bifidum* (or 1 teaspoon each powder), along with 1 teaspoon *L. bulgaricus* powder mixed in 6 to 8 ounces unchilled filtered water, two times daily, for 14 days.

- Instead of the above regimen, take 2 combination capsules that contain all three super strains in an oil-matrix carrier, two times daily, for 14 days.

- In addition to either of the above daily oral regimens, use a yogurt douche to help alleviate the burning and itching of urinary tract infection. To 8 ounces of "true" plain yogurt from your local health food store, add ½ teaspoon each *L acidophilus* powder (NAS or DDS-1 strain) and *L. bulgaricus* powder (LB-51 strain). Use the douche as often as you want to alleviate discomfort. The best time to use it is before bedtime.

- A packaged 14-day program to help alleviate urinary tract infections and vaginitis is available in most health food stores. This product includes vaginal suppositories complete with inserter, and a 14-day supply of high-quality *L. acidophilus* capsules.

- Once the infection has passed, maintain a daily regimen of 1 capsule each of *L. acidophilus* and *B. bifidum* (or ½ teaspoon each powder), along with ½ teaspoon *L. bulgaricus* powder mixed in 6 to 8 ounces unchilled filtered water, three times daily. (Or take 1 combination capsule that contains all three super strains in an oil-matrix carrier, two times daily.)

NOTE: For choosing the highest quality probiotics, see guidelines beginning on page 137.

Vaginitis.

The most common cause of vaginitis—an inflammation of the mucous membranes that line the vagina—is a bacterial or fungal infection. Other causes include radiation therapy, hormonal changes, and irritation from deodorant sprays or douches. Poor personal hygiene is another contributing factor to bacterial and fungal growth.

Abnormal vaginal discharge—one that occurs in large quantities and is malodorous—is the most common symptom of vaginitis. It is generally accompanied by itching, pain, and soreness.

American researchers have shown that the daily supplementation of an *L. acidophilus* strain that produces hydrogen peroxide protects the vaginal tract from yeast or bacterial overgrowth. Using a yogurt douche has long been a proven strategy for treating vaginal itch and irritation. This folk remedy has endured over the years because it works; however, the yogurt must contain high-potency live probiotic cultures. Do not use commercially processed yogurt found on supermarket shelves. (Most of these yogurts do not contain the right *L. bulgaricus* strain.) To prepare the douche, see instructions under Recommended Probiotic Regimen, below.

Direct live culture application brings triple benefits. First, the beneficial bacteria cause rapid displacement of the yeast organisms in the region. Second, they lower pH levels and increase local acidity, which also contributes to yeast die-off. Third, direct application brings welcome symptomatic relief from the burning, itching, and irritation caused by vaginitis.

For more detailed information on the positive effects of probiotics on vaginitis, see the discussion beginning on page 83 in Chapter 7.

RECOMMENDED PROBIOTIC REGIMEN

- If you are diagnosed with vaginitis, take 2 capsules each of *L. acidolphilus* and *B. bifidum* (or 1 teaspoon each powder), along with 1 teaspoon *L. bulgaricus* powder mixed in 6 to 8 ounces unchilled filtered water, two times daily, for 14 days.

- Instead of the above regimen, take 2 combination capsules that contain all three super strains in an oil-matrix carrier, two times daily, for 14 days.

- In addition to either of the above daily oral regimens, use a yogurt douche to help alleviate the burning and itching of vaginitis. To 8 ounces of "true" plain yogurt from your local health food store, add ½ teaspoon each L *acidophilus* powder (NAS or DDS-1 strain) and L. *bulgaricus* powder (LB-51 strain). Use the douche as often as you want to alleviate discomfort. The best time to use it is before bedtime.

- A packaged 14-day program to help alleviate vaginitis and urinary tract infections is available in most health food stores. This product includes vaginal suppositories complete with inserter, and a 14-day supply of high-quality L. *acidophilus* capsules.

- Once the infection has passed, maintain a daily regimen of 1 capsule each of L. *acidophilus* and B. *bifidum* (or ½ teaspoon each powder), along with ½ teaspoon L. *bulgaricus* powder mixed in 6 to 8 ounces unchilled filtered water, three times daily. (Or take 1 combination capsule that contains all three super strains in an oil-matrix carrier, two times daily.)

Note: For choosing the highest quality probiotics, see guidelines beginning on page 137.

Yeast Infection.

See Candidiasis.

A Final Word

The concept of using both traditional and newly emerging treatments for health care is burgeoning throughout North America. It is growing because people are learning to take charge of their own well being. I hope you have found this book to be helpful in your quest to learn more about the vital role that probiotics can play in your life. It is wise, however, always to keep an open mind and to continually learn as much as you can about the health topics that are important to you.

If, after reading this book, you have any questions or comments regarding the use of probiotic supplements, or if you need help in identifying the highest-quality, most-effective probiotic products, please visit me at my website at:

http://www.natren.com
and go to "Ask Natasha"

You can also write to me in care of the publisher:

Natasha Trenev
c/o Avery Publishing Group
120 Old Broadway
Garden City Park, NY 11040

Glossary

acidophilin. A natural antibiotic substance extracted from DDS-1 super strain of *L. acidophilus* (when exclusively grown on milk as per published data).

antibiotic. A substance that kills or inhibits the growth of living microorganisms, especially bacteria, that are found in the gastrointestinal tract. From the Greek: "anti," (against) and "biotics" (life).

bacteria. Single-celled microorganisms that can be either "friendly" or cause disease. Friendly bacteria are normally present in the body and protect it from harmful invading organisms.

benign. This term, which literally means "harmless,"commonly refers to tumors that are not cancerous (malignant).

bifidobacteria. Friendly bacteria that are naturally present in and guard the large intestine.

bifidogenic diet. A diet that includes a high intake of complex carbohydrates (vegetables, fruits, and grains), which encourages high levels of friendly bifidobacteria in the large intestines.

bioavailability. The form in which nutrients can be broken down by the body and metabolized into easily-absorbed components.

chorioamnionitis. Inflammation of the amniotic sac protecting the fetus. Caused by organisms in the fluid surrounding the fetus in the amniotic sac.

fungicide. A chemical agent that destroys or inhibits the growth of fungus. Can be drug or herbal in nature.

Herxheimer Reaction. Temporary toxic or allergic symptoms such as bloating, gas, and/or headaches, that may occur following the onset of a probiotic regimen. This reaction is the result of a massive die-off of harmful bacteria or fungi. It is considered part of the healing process.

in vitro. An experiment that is conducted in an artificial environment, such as a test tube or petri dish.

in vivo. An experiment that is conducted within a living organism— either a lab animal or a human being.

kefir. A creamy drink made from the fermented milk of cows, goats, or sheep. The culture used to make kefir contains a combination of yeast and two strains of lactobacilli.

kumiss. The fermented milk of a mare or camel.

lactase. An enzyme that digests lactose—a sugar found in milk. Lactase is produced by certain strains of lactobacteria (lactobacilli).

Lactobacillus acidophilus. Friendly bacteria that are naturally present in and guard the small intestine.

Lactobacillus bulgaricus. Friendly "transient" bacteria found in yogurt. As *Lactobacillus bulgaricus* passes through the body, it aids the activity of *Lactobacillus acidophilus* and *Bifidobacteria bifidum*.

lactose. Sugar present in milk.

malignant. Term used to refer to cells or groups of cells that are cancerous.

peristalsis. The rhythmic, wave-like muscular activity of the intestines that helps move along digested food.

pH. The abbreviation for hydrogen potential, pH measures acidity levels. A pH level of 7 indicates a neutral environment. Any pH number above 7 signifies an alkaline environment, while numbers below 7 indicate an acidic environment.

phagocytes. White blood cells that ingest and destroy dangerous bacteria and other harmful invaders.

probiotics. Refers to the friendly bacteria that live in the gastrointestinal tract. Meaning "pro-life," probiotics are the opposite of antibiotics. Probiotic supplements are most effective when taken daily as a preventive measure against illness.

supernatant. The growth base for bacteria that contains beneficial metabolic byproducts, including antimicrobial compounds (such as hydrogen peroxide and acidophilin), vitamins, enzymes, cellular building blocks, antioxidants, and immunostimulants.

zone of inhibition. The area in a petri dish that has been cleared of pathogens by a substance being tested. The larger the zone, the greater the inhibitory properties of the test substance.

Bibliography

Abdel-bar, N.M., and N.D. Harris. "Inhibitory effect of *Lactobacillus bulgaricus* on psychotrophic bacteria in associative cultures and in refrigerated foods." *Journal of Food Protection*, 47, 61–64, 1984.

Agel, E.N., B.A. Friend, C.A. Long, and K.M. Shahani. "Bacterial content of raw and processed human milk." *Journal of Food Protection*, 45, No. 6, 533–536, April 1982.

Alm, L., et al. "The effect of acidophilus milk in the treatment of constipation in hospitalized geriatric patients." *XV Symposium*. Swedish Nutrition Foundation, 131–138, 1983.

Alm, Livia. "Effect of fermentation on B vitamin content of milk in Sweden." *Journal of Dairy Science*, 65, 353–359, 1982.

_____. "Effects of fermentation on curd size and digestibility of milk proteins *in vitro* of Swedish fermented products." *Journal of Dairy Science*, 64, 509–514, 1982.

_____. "The effect of *Lactobacillus acidophilus* administration upon the survival of salmonella in randomly selected human carriers." *Prog. Fd. Nutr. Sci.* 7, 13–17, 1983.

Anand, S.K., R.A. Srinivasan, and L.K. Rao. "Antibacterial activity associated with *Bifidobacterium bifidum*." *Cultured Dairy Products Journal*, 19, 6–8, 1984.

Archer, D.L., et al. "Intestinal infection and malnutrition initiate Acquired Immune Deficiency Syndrome (AIDS)." *Nutrition Research* 5, 9–19, 1985.

Ayebo, A.D., I.A. Angelo, and K.M. Shahani. "Effect of ingesting *Lactobacillus acidophilus* milk upon fecal flora and enzyme activity in humans." *Milchwissenschaft*, 35: 730–733, 1980.

Ayebo, A.D., K.M. Shahani, and R. Dam. "Antitumor component(s) of yogurt, I. Fractionation." *Journal of Dairy Science*, 6, 2318–2324, 1981.

Batishh, V.K., H. Chander, and B. Ranjanathan. "Factors affecting enterotoxin production by thermonuclease positive *streptococcus faecium* IF-100 isolated from an infant food." *Journal of Food Science*, 50, 1513–1514, 1985.

Beck, C., and H. Necheles. "Beneficial effects of administration of *Lactobacillus acidophilus* in diarrheal and other intestinal disorders." *American Journal of Gastroenterology*, 35, 522–533, 1961.

Beerens, H., C. Romond, and C. Neut. "Influence of breast feeding on bifido flora of newborn intestine." *American Journal of Clinical Nutrition*, 33, 2434–2439, 1980.

Bellomo, G., et al. "Controlled Double Blind Study of SF68 for Treatment of Diarrhea in Paediatrics." *Current Therapeutics Research*, 28, 827–936, 1980.

————. "New Prospects in the Treatment of Enteritides in Paediatrics." *Medicine et Hygiene*, 37, 3781–3784, 31 October 1979.

Bibek Ray. *Fundamental Food Microbiology*. Boca Raton, FL: CRC Press, Inc., 1996.

Bland, Jeffrey. *Yeast Nutrition Candida albicans: An unsuspected problem*. Nutritional Biochemistry, University of Puget Sound, Tacoma, Washington, 1984.

Bogdanov, I. *Observations on the therapeutic effect of the anti-cancer preparation from Lactobacillus bulgaricus (LB-51) tested on 100 oncological patients*. Laboratory for the Research and Production of Biologically Active Substances, Sofia, Bulgaria, 1982.

Bogdanov, I.G., and P.G. Dalev. "Antitumour glycopeptides from

Lactobacillus bulgaricus cell wall." *FEBS Letters,* 57, 259–261, 1975.

Bolin, Terry, and Rosemary Stanton. *Wind Breaks: Coming to Terms With Flatulence.* New York: Bantam Books, 1993.

Bryant, M. "The shift to probiotics." *Journal of Alternative Medicine,* 6–9, February 1986.

Bullen, C.L., P.V. Tearle, and A.T. Willis. "Bifidobacteria in the intestinal tract of infants: an *in vivo* study." *Journal of Medical Microbiology,* 9, 335–344, 1976.

Butler, B.C., and J.W. Beakley. "Bacterial flora in vaginitis." *American Journal of Obstetrics & Gynecology,* 79, 432–440, 1960.

Camarri, E., et al. "A Double Blind Comparison of Two Different Treatments for Acute Enteritis in Adults." *Chemotherapy,* 27, 466–470, 1981.

Carlson, E. "Enhancement by Candida of *S. aureus, S. marcescens, S. faecalis* in the establishment of infection." *Infection and Immunity,* 39:1, 193–197, January 1983.

Chaitow, Leon. *Candida Albicans: Could Yeast be Your Problem?* Wellingborough, Northhamptonshire, Great Britain: Thorsons, 1985.

Chaitow, Leon, and Simon Martin. *A World Without AIDS.* Wellingborough, Northhamptonshire, Great Britain: Thorsons, 1988.

Chandan, Ramesh C., ed. *Yogurt: Nutritional and Health Properties.* McLean, Virginia: National Yogurt Association, 1989.

Cogan, T.M., and J.P. Accolas, eds. *Dairy Starter Cultures.* New York: VCH Publishers, Inc., 1996.

Collins, D. "Colon Therapy." *Textbook of Natural Medicine,* Seattle: JBCNM, 1986.

Collins, E.B., and Pamela Hardt. "Inhibition of *Candida albicans* by *Lactobacillus acidophilus.*" *Journal of Dairy Science,* 5, 830–832, May 1980.

Crawford, J.T. "Microbiota of dental plaque, caries, gingival disease, related systemic infections." *Microbiology,* 16th edition. New York: Appletone-Century-Crofts, 1976.

Crooke, William G. *The Yeast Connection*. Jackson, TN: Vintage Books, 1988.

Culbert, Michael. *AIDS: Terror, Truth, Triump*. Bradford Foundation, 1987.

Del Vecchio, Blanco C., et al. "Effect of Treatment with SF68 on the Blood Ammonia Curve Following Protein Loading in Subjects with Hepatic Cirrhosis." *Medicine et Hygiene*, 39, 2237–2389, 1981.

Donovan, P. "Bowel Toxaemia, Permeability and Disease." *Textbook of Natural Medicine*, Seattle: JBCNM, 1986.

Dowson, D. "Colonic Cleansing." *Journal of Alternative and Complementary Medicine*, 31–33, May 1988.

Draser, B.S., and M.J. Hill. *Human Intestinal Flora*. London: Academic Press, 1974.

Dubos, R., and R.W. Schaedler. "Some biological effects of the digestive flora." *American Journal of Medical Sciences*, 265–271, September 1962.

Dubos, Rene. *Man Adapting*. New Haven, CT: Yale University Press, 1976.

Elmer, Gary W., C.M. Surawicz, and L.V. McFarland. "Biotherapeutic Agents. A Neglected Modality for the Treatment and Prevention of Selected Intestinal and Vaginal Infections." *Journal of the American Medical Association*, Volume 275, No. 11, 1996.

Farmer, R.E., K.M. Shahani, and G.V. Reddy. "Inhibitory effect of yogurt components upon proliferation of the ascites tumor cells." *Journal of Dairy Science* 58: 7897(abstract), 1975.

Fermented Milks: Current Research. Syndifrais, Association Internationale des Fabricanents de Yaouts, Paris: John Libbey Eurotext, 1989.

Fernandes, C.F., K.M. Shahani, and M.A. Amer. "Control of diarrhea by lactobacilli." *FEMS Microbiology Reviews*, 46, 343–356, 1987.

_____."Therapeutic role of dietary lactobacilli and lactobacillic fermented dairy products." *Journal of Applied Nutrition*, 40, 32–42, 1988.

Ferreira, C.L., and S.E. Gilliland. "Bacteriocin involved in premature death of *Lactobacillus acidophilus* NCFM during growth at pH 6." *Journal of Dairy Science,* 71, 306–315, 1988.

Finegold, S.M., et al. "Comparative effect of broad spectrum antibiotics on non spore-forming anaerobes and normal bowel flora." *Annals New York Academy of Sciences,* 145, 269–281, 1967.

Finegold, Sydney M., and W. Lance George, eds. *Anaerobic Infections in Humans.* New York: Academic Press, 1989.

Fischer, W.L. *How to Fight Cancer and Win.* Vancouver, Canada: Alive Books, 1987.

Fishbaugh, E. "The colon in relation to chronic arthritis." *American Journal of Surgery,* 7: 561–567, 1929.

Friend, B.A., and K.M. Shahani. "Nutritional and therapeutic aspects of Lactobacilli." *Journal of Applied Nutrition,* 36, 125–153, 1984.

Fuchs, N.K. "What Nobody's Told You Yet About Tainted Meat." *Women's Health Newsletter,* May 1993.

Fuller, R., ed. *Probiotics: The Scientific Bases.* London: Chapman & Hall, 1992.

Ganjam, L.S., W.H. Thornton, Jr., R.T. Marshall, and R.S. MacDonald. "Antiproliferative Effects of Yogurt Fractions Obtained by Membrane Dialysis on Cultured Mammalian Intestinal Cells." *Journal of Dairy Science,* 80: 2325–2329, October 1997.

Giannella, R.A., et al. "Gastric acid barrier to ingested microorganisms in man: studies *in vivo* and *in vitro.*" *Gut,* 13, 251–256, 1972.

Gibson, Glenn R., and George T. MacFarlane, eds. *Human Colonic Bacteria: Role in Nutrition, Physiology, and Pathology,* Boca Raton, FL: CRC Press, 1995.

Gilbert, J.P., et al. "Viricidal effects of lactobacillus and yeast fermentation." *Applied Environmental Microbiology,* 452–458, 1983.

Gilliland, S.E. "Beneficial interrelationships between certain microorganisms and humans: candidate microorganisms for use as dietary adjuncts." *Journal of Food Protection,* 42, 164–167, 1979.

Gilliland, S.E., and M.L. Speck. "Antagonistic action of *Lactobacillus acidophilus* toward intestinal and food borne pathogens in associative cultures." *Journal of Food Protection,* 40, 820–823, 1977.

_____. "Instability of *Lactobacillus acidophilus* in yogurt." *Journal of Dairy Science,* 60, 1394–1398, 1977.

Gilliland, S.E., et al. "Assimilation of cholesterol by *Lactobacillus acidophilus.*" *Applied and Environmental Microbiology,* 377–381, February 1985.

Goldin, B.R., L. Seson, J. Dwyer, M. Sevfon, and L. Gorbach. "Effect of diet and *Lactobacillus acidophilus* supplements on human fecal bacterial enzymes." *National Cancer Institute,* 64, 255–261, 1980.

Gorbach, S.L., T. Chang, and B. Goldin. "Successful treatment of relapsing clostridium difficile colitis with Lactobacillus GG." *Lancet,* 1519, 26 December 1987.

Gracey, M.S. "Nutrition, bacteria, and the gut." *British Medical Bulletin,* 37, No.1, 71–75, 1981.

Grutte, F.K., and W. Muller-Beuthow. "Instability of the normal intestinal flora in human infants." *Human Gastrointestinal Microflora,* 39–44, Leipzig: J.A. Barth, Verlag, 1980.

"Gut ecology and health implications." *Dairy Council Digest,* 50, 13–17, 1979.

Hamdan, I.Y., and E.M. Mikolajcik. "Acidolin: an antibiotic produced by *Lactobacillus acidophilus.*" *Journal of Antibiotics,* 8, 631–636, 1974.

Hangee Bauer, C.S. "Lactobacilli and human health." Seattle, WA: Rounds/Journal Club of the John Bastyr College of Naturopathic Medicine, 1987.

Hansen, Robert. "Bifidobacteria have come to stay." Reprint from *North European Dairy Journal,* No. 3, 2–6, 1985.

Hargrove, R.E., and J.A. Alford. "Growth rate and feed efficiency of rats fed yogurt and other fermented milks." *Journal of Dairy Science,* 61, 11–19, 1978.

Helferich, W.M., and D. Westhoff. *All About Yogurt.* Englewood Cliffs, NJ: Prentice Hall, Inc., 1980.

Hentges, David J., ed. *Human Intestinal Microflora in Health and Disease.* Academic Press, New York: 1983.

Hentges, David J., et al. "Effect of high-beef diet on the fecal bacterial flora of humans." *Cancer Research,* 37, 568–571, 1977.

Hepner, G., et al. "Hypocholesterolemic effect of yogurt and milk." *American Journal of Clinical Nutrition,* 32, 19–24, 1979.

Hoover, Dallas G., and Larry R. Steenson, eds. *Bacteriocins of Lactic Acid Bacteria.* San Diego, CA: Academic Press, 1993.

Huppert, M., et al. "Pathogenesis of *Candida albicans*; I. The effect of antibiotics on the growth of *Candida albicans*." 65, 171–176, Chapel Hill, NC: Department of Bacteriology and Immunology, University of North Carolina School of Medicine, 1953.

Jackson, G.G., and H.F. Dowling. "Adverse effects of antibiotic treatment." *G.P.,* 34–40, August 1953.

Jameson, R.M. "The prevention of recurrent urinary tract infection in women." *The Practitioner,* 216, 178–181, 1976.

Kageyama, T., et al. "The effect of bifidobacterium administration in patients with leukemia." *Bifidobacteria Microflora,* 3, 29–33, 1984.

Kantor, J., et al. "Colon Studies cecal stasis; its significance to proximal colon stasis." *American Journal of Roentgenology and Radium Therapy,* 24 (1), 1–20, 1930.

Kay, H.W., and W. Heeschen. "Antileukemic effects in mice from fermentation products of *Lactobacillus bulgaricus*." *Milchwissenschaft,* 38, 257–260, 1983.

Kilara, A., and K.M. Shahani. "Effect of cryoprotective agents on freeze-drying and storage of lactic cultures." *Cultured Dairy Products Journal,* 11, 5, 8–11, 1976.

_____. "Lactic fermentations of dairy foods and their biological significance." *Journal of Dairy Science,* 61, 1793–1800, 1987.

Kim, H.S. "Characterization of lactobacilli and bifidobacteria fats applied to dietary adjuncts." *Cultured Dairy Products Journal,* 6–9, August 1988.

Kim, J.S., and S.E. Gilliland. "*Lactobacillus acidophilus* as a dietary adjunct for milk to aid lactose digestion in humans." *Journal of Dairy Science*, 66, 959–966, 1983.

Klebanoff, S.J., and R.W. Coombs. "Viricidal Effect of *Lactobacillus acidophilus* on Human Immunodeficiency Virus Type 1: Possible Role in Heterosexual Transmission." *The Rockefeller University Press Journal*, Vol. 174, 289–292, July 1991.

Lappe, Marc. *When Antibiotics Fail: Restoring the Ecology of the Body*. Berkeley, CA: North Atlantic Books, 1986.

Law, B.A., and M.E. Sharpe. "Streptococci in the dairy industry." *Streptococci*, 263–278, London: Academic Press, Inc., 1978.

Le-Roith, D., J. Shiloach, J. Roth, and M. Lesniak. "Insulin or a closely related molecule is native to *E. coli*," *Journal Biol-Chemistry*, 256: 6533–6536, 1981.

"Les Laits Fermentes (Fermented Milks)," Congress International. Paris: John Libbey Eurotext, 1989.

Levy, Stuart B. *The Antibiotic Paradox: How Miracle Drugs Are Destroying the Miracle*. New York: Plenum Press, 1992.

Mann, G.V., and A. Sperry. "Studies of a surfactant and cholesterolemia in the Masai." *American Journal of Clinical Nutrition*, 27, 464–469, 1974.

Mao, Yilei, et al. "The Effects of *Lactobacillus* Strains and Oat Fiber on Methotrexate Induced Enterocolitis in Rats." *Gastroenterology*, III: 334–344, 1996.

Marshall, H., and C. Thomson. "Colon irrigation in the treatment of mental disease." *New England Journal of Medicine*, 207: 454–457, 1932.

Matalon, M.E., and W.E. Sandine. "*Lactobacillus bulgaricus, Streptococcus thermophilus* and yogurt: a review." *Cultured Dairy Products Journal*, 6–11, November 1986.

McCann, Michael L. "Reflorastation Therapy for Inflammatory Bowel Diseases (IBD), Both Crohn's (CD) and Ulcerative Colitis (UC)." *Journal Allergy Clinical Immunology*, 359, January 1993.

_____. "Treatment of Ulcerative Colitis (UC) and Crohn's Disease

(CD) by Gut Microflora Replacement after Antimicrobial Decontamination." Parma, OH: Parma Medical Center, 1991.

McCann, Michael L., R.S. Abrams, and R.P. Nelson. "Recolonization Therapy with Nonadhesive *Escherichia coli* for Treatment of Inflammatory Bowel Disease, Microbial Pathogenesis, and Immune Response." *Annals of the New York Academy of Sciences*, Volume 730, 243–245, 1994.

McCann, Michael L., R. Greinwald, U. Sonnenborn, R. Nelson, and R.A. Good. "Long Lasting Remissions of Inflammatory Bowel Disease Produced by Sustained Recolonization with Nonpathogenic *E. coli*." *American Academy of Allergy and Immunology*, October 1991

McCann, Michael L., and Paul Jaconella. "Bowel Flora Recolonization Therapy in Ankylosing Spondylitis." Fifth Annual Conference on Clinical Immunology, 1993.

McCann, Michael L., R.P. Nelson, and R.A. Good. "Clinical Recovery in Inflammatory Bowel Disease (IBD) Following Bowel Flora Replacement with *E. coli*." Fifth Annual Conference on Clinical Immunology, 1990.

Metchnickoff, E. *The Prolongation of Life*. New York: G.P. Putnam & Sons, 1908.

Mikolajcik, E.M., and I.Y. Hamdan. "*Lactobacillus acidophilus*, II. Antimicrobial agents." *Cultured Dairy Products Journal*, 18–20, February 1975.

Mindell, Earl. *Unsafe at Any Meal*. New York: Warner Books, 1987.

Moroni, M. *Vecchi E. Nuovi Orientamenti nel rattamento delle enteriti Medico epaziente*, Vol. 6, March, 1979.

Mott, G.E., et al. "Lowering of serum cholesterol by intestinal bacteria in cholesterol-fed piglets." *Lipids*, 8, 428–431, 1973.

Muting, D., et al. "The effect of bacterium bifidum on intestinal bacterial flora and toxic protein metabolites in chronic liver disease." *American Journal of Proctology*, 19, 336–342, 1968.

Nankaya, R. "Role of bifidobacteria in enteric infection." *Bifidobacteria Microflora*, 5, 51–55, 1984.

Nikolov, N.M. "Acidophilus paste, Bulgarian yogurt, and other cultured milk products." Sofia, Bulgaria: Zemizdat, 1962.

Okamura, N., et al. "Interaction of shigella with bifidobacteria." *Bifidobacteria Microflora* 5, 51–55, 1986.

Pabst, M.J., et al. "Cultured human monocytes require exposure to bacterial products to maintain an optimal oxygen radical response." *Journal of Immunology*, 123–128, 1982.

Pearce, J.L., and J.R. Hamilton. "A controlled trial of orally administered lactobacilli in acute infantile diarrhea." *Journal of Pediatrics*, 84, 261–262, 1974.

Perdigon, M.E., et al. "Enhancement of immune response in mice fed with *Streptococcus thermophilus* and *Lactobacillus acidophilus*." *Journal of Dairy Science*, 70, 5, 919–926, 1987.

Pizzorno, J., and M. Murray. *Textbook of Natural Medicine*, Seattle, WA: JBCNM, 1987.

Pollman, D.S., D.M. Danielson, W.B. Wren, E.R. Peo, Jr., and K.M. Shahani. "Influence of *Lactobacillus acidophilus* on gnotobiotic and conventional pigs." *Journal of Animal Science*, 51 (3), 629–637, 1980.

Porubcan, et al. "Preparation of culture concentrates for direct vat set cheese production." United States Government Patent 4,115,119, September 19, 1978.

Poupard, J.A., I. Husain, and R.F. Norris. "Biology of the Bifidobacteria." *Bacteriological Reviews*, 37, 2, 136–165, June 1973.

Quinn, T.C. "Gay bowel syndrome, the broadened spectrum of non-genital infection." *Postgraduate Medicine*, 76, 197–210, 1984.

Rao, D.R., and K.M. Shahani. "Vitamin content of cultured milk products." *Cultured Dairy Products Journal*, 6–10, February 1987.

Rapoport, L., and W.I. Levine. "Treatment of oral ulceration with lactobacillus tablets." *Oral Surgery, Oral Medicine, and Oral Pathology*, 20, 591–593, 1965.

Rasic, Jeremija, Istevan Klem, Dusan Jovanovic, and Ac Mira. "Antimicrobial effect of *Lactobacillus acidophilus* and *Lactobacillus delbrueckii* susbp. *bulgaricus* against *Helicobacter pylori* in vitro." *Arch.*

Gastroenterohepatol, (No. 1), 158–160, 1995.

Rasic, J.L. "Nutritive value of yogurt." *Cultured Dairy Products Journal,* 6–9, August 1987.

————. "Occurrence of *B. infantis* and *B. bifidum* in the gut of infants and adults." Letter of correspondence, 1988.

————. "The role of dairy foods containing bifido and acidophilus bacteria in nutrition and health." *North European Dairy Journal,* 4, 80–88, 1983.

Rasic, J.L., and J.A. Kurmann. *Bifidobacteria and Their Role,* Boston: Birkhauser Verlag, 1983.

————. *Yoghurt: Scientific Grounds, Technology, Manufacture and Preparation.* Switzerland, 1978.

Reddy, G.V., et al. "Antitumour activity of yogurt components." *Journal of Food Protection,* 46, 8–11, 1983.

Reddy, G.V., K.M. Shahani, B.A. Friend, and R.C. Chandan. "Natural antibiotic activity of *L. acidophilus* and *bulgaricus.*" *Cultured Dairy Products,* 18, 2, 15–19, 1983.

Rhoads, J.L., et al. "Chronic vaginal candidiasis in women with human immunodeficiency virus infection." *JAMA,* 257, 3105–3107, 1987.

Riise, T. "The probiotic concept—a review." *Chris Hansen's Laboratory,* Copenhagen, Denmark, 1–8, June 1981.

Robbins-Browne, R.M., and M.M. Levine. "The fate of ingested lacto-bacilli in the proximal small intestine." *American Journal of Clinical Nutrition,* 34, 514–519, 1981.

Robinson, R.K., ed. *Therapeutic Properties of Fermented Milks,* New York: Elsevier Science Publishers, LTD, 1991.

Rowland, I.R., and P. Grasso. "Degradation of N-Nitrosamines by intestinal bacteria." *Applied Microbiology,* Vol. 29, No. 1, 7–12, January 1975.

Savage, D.C. "Factors influencing biocontrol of bacterial pathogens in the intestines." *Food Technology,* 82–87, July 1987.

Schardt, D.,and S. Schmidt. "Fishing for Safe Seafood." *Nutritional Action Health Letter*, 1, 3–5, November 1996.

Schecter, A., J. Ryan, and J. Constable. "Polychlorinated PCDD and PCDF in human breast milk from Vietnam compared with cow's milk and human milk from North American Continent." *Chemosphere*, 16, 2003–2016, 1987.

Schecter, A., and T. Gasiewicz. "Human breast milk levels of dioxins and dibenzofurans: Significance with respect to current risks."*Solving Hazardous Waste Problems*, Washington, DC: American Chemical Society, 1987.

_____. "Health hazard assessment of chlorinated dioxins and dibenzofurans contained in human milk." *Chemosphere*, 16, 2147–2154, 1987.

Schrag, Ludvig, and Heinz Singer. *The Calf Book*. Hengersberg, Germany: Schober Verlags–GMBH, 1992.

Schuster, George S., ed. *Oral Microbiology and Infectious Disease*. Baltimore, MD: Williams & Wilkins, 1983.

Seaman, B. *Women and the Crisis in Sex Hormones*. Harvester Press, 1978.

Shahani, K.M. "Antiviral and antifungal effect of lactobacilli." *The New Show Daily*, July 12, 1987.

Shahani, K.M., and A.D. Ayebo. "Role of dietary lactobacilli in gastrointestinal microecology." *American Journal of Clinical Nutrition*, 33, 2248–2257, November 1980.

Shahani, K.M., and R.C. Chandan. "Nutritional and healthful aspects of cultured and culture-containing dairy products." *Journal of Dairy Science*, 62, 1685–1694, 1979.

Shahani, K.M., and B.A. Friend. "Nutritional and therapeutic aspects of Lactobacilli." *Journal of Applied Nutrition*, 37, 2, 136–165, June 1973.

Shahani, K.M., G.V. Reddy, and A.M. Joe. "Nutritional and Therapeutic aspects of cultured dairy products." Proc XIX, International Dairy Congress, Ie, 569–570, 1974.

Shahani, K.M., and Jayantkumar R. Vakil. "Antibiotic acidophilus and process of preparing the same." United States Patent No. 3, 689, 640, 5 September 1972.

Shahani, K.M., J.R. Vakil, and A. Kilara. "Natural antibiotic activity of *Lactobacillus acidophilus* and *bulgaricus* II. Isolation of acidophilin from *L. acidophilus*." *Cultured Dairy Products Journal*, 12, 2, 8–11, 1977.

Shahani, K.M., et al. "Role and significance of enzymes in human milk." *American Journal of Clinical Nutrition*, 33, 1861–1868, 1980.

Simon, G.L., and S.L. Gorbach. "Intestinal flora in health and disease." *Physiology of the Gastrointestinal Tract*, L.R. Johnson, ed. New York: Raven Press, 1981.

Siver, R.H. "Lactobacillus for the control of acne." *Journal of the Medical Society of New Jersey*, 58, 52–83, 1964.

Sneath, P.H.A. *Bergey's Manual of Systematic Bacteriology*, Vol. 2, Baltimore, MD: Williams & Wilkins, 1986.

Socransky, S.S. "Bacteriological studies of developing supragingival dental plaque." *J. Periodontal Res.* 12, 90–106, 1977.

Speck, M.L. "Contributions of microorganisms to food and nutrition." *Nutrition News*, 38, 4, 13, December 1975.

_____."Interactions among lactobacilli and Man." *Journal of Dairy Science*, 59, 338–343, 1975.

Stein, Jay, ed. *Internal Medicine*. Boston: Little, Brown and Company, Inc., 1983.

Thompson, L.U., J.A. David, M.A. Jenkins, V. Amer, et al. "The effect of fermented and unfermented milks on serum cholesterol." *American Journal of Clinical Nutrition*, 36, 11, 6, 111, December 1982.

Timms, Moira, and Zacharia Zar. *Natural Sources*. CA: Celestial Arts, 1978.

Trenev, Natasha. "Doctor's Guide: Probiotics and Candidiasis." *The American Chiropractor*, February 1989.

_____. "Our Intestinal Dilemma." *Alive Magazine*, January 1991.

_____. "The Scientific Criteria for Selecting Efficacious Probiotics."

International Journal of Alternative & Complementary Medicine, 1189–1206, April 1994.

_____. "Take Acidophilus With You When Traveling Out of Area." *Food for Health,* Vol. 3, No. 6, 1991.

_____. "You Need Bifidobacteria More Than Ever." *The American Chiropractor,* 74–75, August 1988.

Trenev, N., and J. Rasic. "Advances in Food Science—Probiotics and the Role of Probiotics in Modern Nutrition," and "Geriatric and Infant Nutrition." Two abstracts accepted for publication and oral presentation at the XV International Congress of Nutrition in Adelaide, Australia, 1993.

Truss, C. Orion. *The Missing Diagnosis.* PO Box 26508, Birmingham, AL, 35226, 1983 and 1986.

_____. "The Role of *Candida albicans* in Human Illness." *Orthomolecular Psychiatry,* Vol. 10, No. 4, 228–238, 1981.

Vos, J.G. "Immune suppression as related to toxicology." *CRC Critical Reviews in Toxicology,* Vol. 5, 67–101, 1977.

Warshaw, A., C. Bellini, and W. Walker. "The intestinal mucosal barrier to intact antigen protein." *American Journal of Surgery,* 133: 55–58, 1977.

Warshaw, A., W. Walker, and K. Isselbacher. "Protein uptake in the intestines; Evidence of intact macromolecules." *Gastroenterology,* 66: 987–992, 1974.

Warshaw, A., W. Walker, W. Cornell, and K. Isselbacher. "Small intestine permeability to macromolecules." *Lab. Invest.,* 25: 675–684, 1971.

Walker, Allan W., and Kurt J. Isselbacher. "Uptake and Transport of Macro molecules by the Intestine: Possible role in clinical disorder." *Gastroenterology,* 67: 531–550, 1974.

Weekes, D.J. "Management of Herpes Simplex with a virostatic bacterial agent." *E.E.N.T. Digest,* 25, 1983.

Werbach, Melvyn. *Nutritional Influences on Illness.* Wellingborough, England: Thorsons, 1989.

Wexler, Hannah. "Microbiology of Obstetric and Gynecologic Infections." *Pharmanual: The role of piperacillin/tazobactam in the treatment of obstetric and gynecological infections*, Montreal, Quebec, Canada: PhamraLibti Publishers, Inc., 1994.

Wheater, D.M., et al. "Possible identity of 'Lactobacillin' with hydrogen peroxide produced by Lactobacilli." *Nature*, 170, 623–624, 1952.

Williams, E., and W. Hemmings. "Intestinal uptake and transport of proteins in the adult rat." *Proceedings of the Royal Society of London*, 203: 177–189, 1979.

Zaika, L.L., et al. "Inhibition of lactic acid bacteria by herbs." *Journal of Food Science*, 48, 1455–1459, 1983.

Index

B

B-complex vitamins, 45–47
Babies, unborn, and bacteria,
  55–58
Baby bacteria. *See Bifidobacteria
  infantis.*
Bacteria, beneficial
  antibiotic action of, 73–87
  in the birth canal, 56, 57
  cancer-fighting, 100–102
  cholesterol-fighting, 48
  classification of, 35–37
  culturing, 121–122
  and the immune system,
    102–103
  and nutrition, 39–40
  and weight control, 47–48
Bacteria, beneficial, foes of
  anal intercourse, 69
  antacids, 66
  antibiotics, 69–71
  bacterial interaction, hostile, 67
  laxatives, 66–67
  poor diet, 68–69
  reduced estrogen levels,
    71–72
Bacterial count of probiotic
  supplements, 125
Bacterial infections and the
  unborn child, 55–58
Bacterial interaction, harmful, 67
Bacterial vaginosis, 56–58
Bamboo spine. *See* Ankylosing
  spondylitis.
Batish, Dr. V.K., 63
Beakley, J.W., 84
Beerens, Dr. H., 61

Bifidobacteria, 4, 35, 78–79,
  117–118
Bifidobacteria infantis, 58, 61–62
Bifidobacteria bifidum Malyoth
  super strain, 118
Bifidobacteria infantis NLS super
  strain, 118–120
Bifidobacteria and Their Role, 210
Big Three Trio probiotic
  supplement, 129
Bile, 22, 48, 50
Bioavailability, definition of, 39
Biotin, 155–156
Birth control, effects of, 72
Bland, Jeffrey, 157
Bogdanov, Dr. Ivan, 106–107,
  120
Botulism. *See* Food Poisoning.
Bowel toxicity. *See* Toxic bowel.
Breast milk, bacteria in, 58–60,
  61
Bryant, Monica, 188
Butler, B.C., 84

C

Calcium, bioavailability of,
  41–42
Calcium and osteoporosis, 195
Caloric intake, determining,
  24–25
Cancer. *See also* Radiation
  sickness.
  cancer-fighting bacteria,
    100–102
  effects of diet on, 99–100
  risks, reducing, 99
  warning signs of, 98

Journal of Food Science, The, 63
Journal of Infectious Diseases, The, 85
Journal of the New York Academy of Sciences, 164

K

Kefir, 11
Klebanoff, S.J., 85, 95–96
Klebsiella, 143–144
Kumiss, 10–11
Kurmann, Dr. J.A., 210

L

Lactase, 33
Lactic acid, 33
Lactobacilli, antiviral action of, 92–93
  on herpesvirus, 93–95
  on HIV virus and AIDS, 95–96
Lactobacillus acidophilus, 4, 32–33
  and the immune system, 103
  and reduction of cholesterol, 50–51
  as a cancer fighting agent, 100–101
  DDS-1 super strain, 115–117
  NAS super adhesion strain, 117
  in probiotic supplements, 114
  effects on vaginitis, 83–87
Lactobacillus bulgaricus, 5, 15, 32–33, 76–77, 120
  LB-51 super strain, 120

Lactobacillus casei, 32
Lactose intolerance, 40–41, 192–194
Lactulose, 210–211
Large intestine
  bacteria inhabiting, 34–35
  function of, 25–26
Laxatives, effects of, 66–67
Le Roith, Dr. D., 168
Lesniak, Dr. M., 168
Leukemia, 97
Levine, Dr. W.I., 94–95
Listeria bacteria, 175–176
Listeriosis, 175–176
Liver, function of, 22
Low-density lipoproteins (LDLs), 48–49
Lymphoma, 97
Lyophilization. *See* Freeze-drying.

M

Masai tribesmen, 49
McCann, Dr. Michael L., 164
Medical Hypotheses, 96
Metchnikoff, Dr. Elie, 9–10
Migraine headache. *See* Headache.
Mikolajcik, E.M., 74, 92–93
Minerals, processing, 25
Mouth
  bacteria inhabiting, 30
  function of, 20
Mouth sores. *See* Canker sores; Cold sores.
Mucous colitis. *See* Irritable bowel syndrome.

Y

Z

What You Don't Know About Food Can Hurt You

GUESS WHAT CAME TO DINNER

PARASITES AND YOUR HEALTH

Ann Louise Gittleman

FROM THE BEST-SELLING AUTHOR OF *BEYOND PRITIKIN*

0-89529-570-9 • $9.95

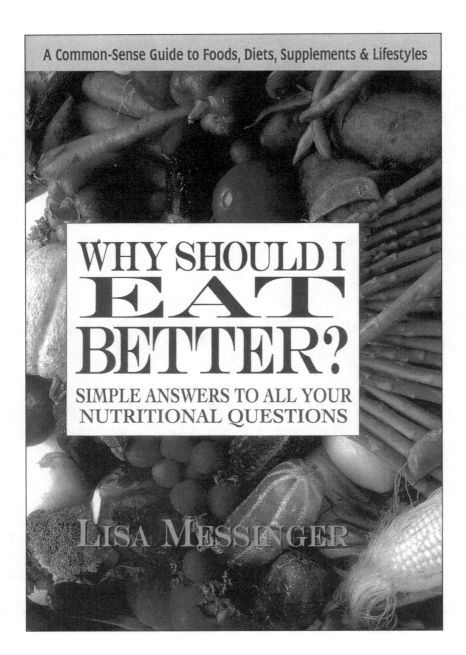

A Common-Sense Guide to Foods, Diets, Supplements & Lifestyles

WHY SHOULD I EAT BETTER?

SIMPLE ANSWERS TO ALL YOUR NUTRITIONAL QUESTIONS

LISA MESSINGER

0-89529-508-3 • $9.95

REVISED AND EXPANDED

A COMPREHENSIVE & UP-TO-DATE
SELF-HELP APPROACH TO GOOD HEALTH

Prescription for

NUTRITIONAL HEALING

SECOND EDITION

A PRACTICAL A–Z REFERENCE TO
DRUG-FREE REMEDIES USING VITAMINS,
MINERALS, HERBS & FOOD SUPPLEMENTS

JAMES F. BALCH, M.D. • PHYLLIS A. BALCH, C.N.C.

0-89529-727-2 • $19.95

A GUIDE TO OVERCOMING THE DISCOMFORTS
OF INDIGESTION USING DRUG-FREE REMEDIES

Heartburn

OVERCOME NAUSEA • BLOATEDNESS • DISTRESS •

And What To

ACIDITY • QUEASINESS • GAS • STOMACH PAIN •

Do About It

INTESTINAL CRAMPS • GASTRITIS • BURNING

Dr. James F. Balch
BEST-SELLING COAUTHOR OF *PRESCRIPTION FOR NUTRITIONAL HEALING*

Dr. Morton Walker
BEST-SELLING COAUTHOR OF *HYPERBARIC OXYGEN THERAPY*

0-89529-792-2 • $10.95

Healthy Habits
are easy to come by—
IF YOU KNOW WHERE TO LOOK!

Get the latest information on:
- **better health • diet & weight loss**
- **the latest nutritional supplements**
- **herbal healing • homeopathy and more**

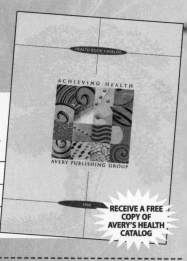

COMPLETE AND RETURN THIS CARD RIGHT AWAY!

Where did you purchase this book?
- ❑ bookstore
- ❑ supermarket
- ❑ health food store
- ❑ other (please specify)_____
- ❑ pharmacy

Name_____

Street Address_____

City_____ State_____ Zip_____

RECEIVE A FREE COPY OF AVERY'S HEALTH CATALOG

GIVE ONE TO A FRIEND ...

Healthy Habits
are easy to come by—
IF YOU KNOW WHERE TO LOOK!

Get the latest information on:
- **better health • diet & weight loss**
- **the latest nutritional supplements**
- **herbal healing • homeopathy and more**

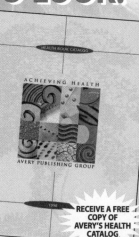

COMPLETE AND RETURN THIS CARD RIGHT AWAY!

Where did you purchase this book?
- ❑ bookstore
- ❑ supermarket
- ❑ health food store
- ❑ other (please specify)_____
- ❑ pharmacy

Name_____

Street Address_____

City_____ State_____ Zip_____

RECEIVE A FREE COPY OF AVERY'S HEALTH CATALOG

Avery Publishing Group
120 Old Broadway
Garden City Park, NY 11040

DISCARD

Avery Publishing Group
120 Old Broadway
Garden City Park, NY 11040